THE COMPLETE GUIDE TO
BACK REHABILITATION

THE COMPLETE GUIDE TO
BACK REHABILITATION

Dr Christopher M. Norris

BLOOMSBURY

LONDON · NEW DELHI · NEW YORK · SYDNEY

Bloomsbury Sport
An imprint of Bloomsbury Publishing Plc

50 Bedford Square	1385 Broadway
London	New York
WC1B 3DP	NY 10018
UK	USA

www.bloomsbury.com

BLOOMSBURY and the Diana logo are trademarks of Bloomsbury Publishing Plc

First published 2015

British Library Cataloguing-in-Publication Data.
A catalogue record for this book is available from the British Library.

Library of Congress Cataloguing-in-Publication data has been applied for.

ISBN: PB: 978-1-4081-8722-7
 ePDF: 978-1-4729-1672-3
 ePub: 978-1-4729-1671-6

10 9 8 7 6 5 4 3 2 1

Typeset in Adobe Caslon by seagulls.net
Printed and bound in China by Toppan Leefung Printing

Bloomsbury Publishing Plc makes every effort to ensure that the papers used in the manufacture of our books are natural, recyclable products made from wood grown in well-managed forests. Our manufacturing processes conform to the environmental regulations of the country of origin.

To find out more about our authors and books visit www.bloomsbury.com. Here you will find extracts, author interviews, details of forthcoming events and the option to sign up for our newsletters.

CONTENTS

HOW THE BACK WORKS

GENERAL DESCRIPTION

The spine is divided into five regions: cervical (neck), thoracic (mid-) and lumbar (lower), with the sacrum and coccyx forming the rudiments of the tail. The spinal column as a whole is made up of 33 individual bones (vertebrae). Each vertebra is numbered to show its position. Cervical vertebra numbers start with 'C', thoracic 'T', lumbar 'L' and sacral 'S'. So, for example, the second cervical vertebra counting down from the head is C2, and the fourth C4. The numbering system for every section begins at the head, so the last lumbar vertebra is L5. Note also that, until the 1950s, the Thoracic area was commonly called the Dorsal region, so old books or papers which quote them may use 'D' instead of the 'T' to denote this region. In addition to this, some traditional exercise organisations still use the term 'Dorsal' in their teaching.

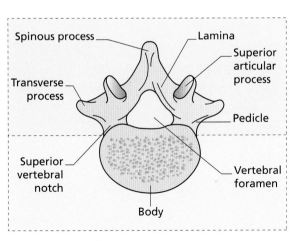

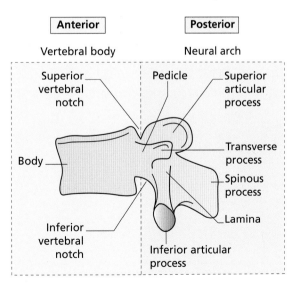

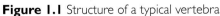

Figure 1.1 Structure of a typical vertebra

STRUCTURE OF A TYPICAL VERTEBRA

A typical vertebra (see fig. 1.1) has an anterior (front) and posterior (back) part. The anterior portion consists of a large circular body flattened slightly at its back. This body is attached above and below to a spongy vertebral disc. The posterior portion of the vertebra forms an arch (called a neural or vertebral arch). This has a total of seven processes attached to it.

At the back of the vertebra is the *spinous process*, the tip of which can be felt with the fingers (this is made easier if the subject bends forward so that the skin is stretched tight). Jutting out at the sides are two *transverse processes*.

These form the attachment of muscles and are located approximately two finger widths from the centre line. They are covered by muscle and are thus harder to palpate (palpation is the practice of using one's hands to examine organs or other parts of the body). However, deep palpation can usually locate the transverse processes on a very lean subject. Just in front of the vertebral body is a hole called the *vertebral foramen*, which encloses the spinal canal. At the angle between the spinous process and transverse process is a shallow cup called the *articular process,* and there are four of these, two on each side, one above (superior) and one below (inferior). Each articular process is cup shaped and connects with a similar cup of the vertebra above and below to form a small flat joint on each side of the vertebra called a *facet joint* (also known as an apophyseal joint). The point at which the neural arch attaches to the vertebral body is called the *pedicle* and the point of attachment to the spinous process is called the *lamina*.

Definition

A process is a projection of bone that juts through the skin to form a small mound or knobble on the skin surface. Examples are found on several bones including vertebrae (spinous process), the radius (styloid process), and temporal bone of the jaw (mastoid process).

Definition

The spinal canal is the space in the vertebrae, enclosed by the vertebral foramen, through which the spinal cord passes.

Clinical note

In a operation called a Laminectomy a small piece of bone along the lamina is removed to provide more space around the notes. The operation is performed in cases of disc prolapse (slipped disc) and spinal stenosis (narrowing of the spinal canal). Laminectomy is a microsurgery procedure and often some ligament and other tissue will be removed at the same time.

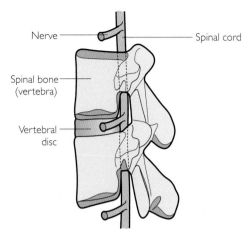

Figure 1.2 Spinal segment

Each pair of spinal bones together forms a single unit called a spinal segment (see fig. 1.2). As we have seen there are three main joints to each vertebra: the spinal disc in the centre and a small facet joint at each side. The disc is fibrous, while the facet joints contain fluid. We will see in chapter 2 how these joints can be injured or affected by medical conditions.

> **Definition**
> A synovial joint is the most common movable joint in the human body. It consists of two bone ends covered by cartilage (hyaline cartilage). The joint is contained within a fibrous bag called the joint capsule, which is lined by a synovial membrane. The joint is lubricated by synovial fluid.

REGIONAL DIFFERENCES

Figure 1.3 shows the differences in structure of typical vertebrae from each spinal region. The cervical vertebra has a small hole at each side called

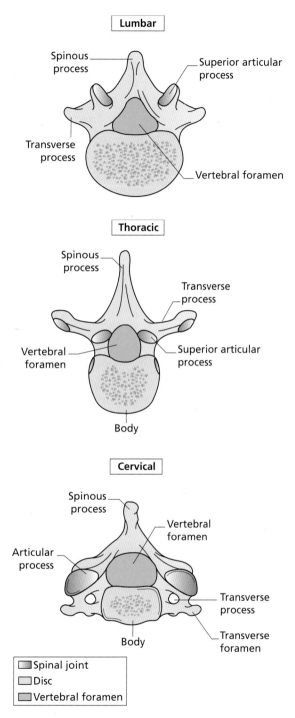

Figure 1.3 Differences in structure between typical vertebrae in each spinal region

the *transverse foramen* for the passage of the verte-bral arteries through the neck into the brain. The thoracic vertebrae have small joints for the attach-ment of the ribs (see fig. 1.4). The lumbar verte-brae are large, strong bones covered with powerful muscles. They bear the whole weight of the trunk above them, hence the slightly stubby appearance of their spinous and transverse processes.

CERVICAL REGION

The cervical region is subdivided into two func-tional parts. The upper portion directly below the head is called the *sub-occipital region* (the occiput being the lower back portion of the skull). The C1 and C2 bones make up this region and these two bones are intimately connected with skull movements – especially nodding actions. The lower portion of the neck is called the *lower cervi-cal region* and takes in the bones C3 to C7. This region is more involved with twisting (rotation) and side bending (lateral flexion) actions.

As mentioned above, one of the unique features of the cervical vertebrae is the presence of the vertebral arteries, which pass through the vertebral foramina within the transverse processes. Because the first cervical vertebra (C1) does not have a transverse process, these arteries travel behind the arch of the vertebra, and in 7.5 per cent of people the arteries also do so in C7. The vertebral arteries supply blood to the rear part of the brain. Damage to the arteries can occur during a neck injury, and they can be compressed or restricted in chronic neck conditions and in cases of *atherosclerosis*.

Reduction of the blood flow through the arter-ies to the brain is called *vertebrobasilar insufficiency* or VBI (also known as vertebral artery insuf-ficiency). One of the most common mechanical causes of this condition is prolonged neck exten-

Definition
Flexion refers to the action of bending or being in a bent position.

Definition
Atherosclerosis is a thickening or hardening of an artery wall due to the build up of fatty plaques.

sion over a period of some minutes, which can in extreme cases lead to a stroke.

THORACIC REGION

In the chest region the thoracic vertebrae are attached to the ribs by two joints: the costover-tebral (CV) joint between vertebral body and the rib, and the costotransverse (CT) joint between the transverse process at the side of the vertebra and the rib angle, where the rib curves to form the drum of the chest (see fig. 1.4). When looking at someone's back, the spinous processes are in the middle forming a straight column of bumps. The CV joint is about two finger breadths to the side lying in the furrow of the back (*paraspinal gutter*). The CT joint is about 3 finger breadths to the side, covered by the large erector spinae muscles.

Key point
In the thoracic spine, the spinous process is in the centre of the back, the costovertebral joint slightly out to the side, and the costotransverse joint further out still.

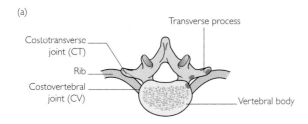

(a)

Costotransverse joint (CT)

Rib

Costovertebral joint (CV)

Transverse process

Vertebral body

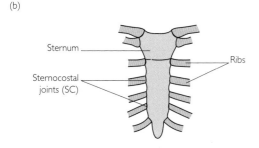

(b)

Sternum

Sternocostal joints (SC)

Ribs

Figure 1.4 Joints between the ribs and thoracic spine

LUMBAR REGION

Movement of the lumbar vertebrae is intimately linked to that of the pelvis, as well as the upper spine. The upper portion of the lumbar spine (L1 and L2) moves with the thoracic spine, especially during shoulder blade and ribcage movements. The lower lumbar vertebrae (L3, L4 and L5) move closely with the pelvis, and this combined region is often referred to as the lumbo-pelvis.

THE SACRUM AND PELVIS

At the base of the lumbar spine is the pelvis. This is ring shaped with two large flat bones (*iliac bones*) on each side. These attach at the front through the *pubis* to form the *pubic symphysis* and at the back to the *sacrum*, which forms a keystone between the two. The sacrum is a triangular shaped bone, which together with the thin pointed coccyx forms the remnants of our

> **Key point**
> The sacroiliac joint joins the sacrum to the pelvis. It is often painful during pregnancy and following childbirth.

tail. The sacrum attaches to the iliac bones via the *sacroiliac joint* or SIJ.

These regions are important as there is significant risk of injury, especially during pregnancy and childbirth. The SIJ and pubic symphysis are each filled with fibrous material and normally give little movement. During childbirth, however, the fibrous material softens and the joint moves to allow the pelvis to expand. This motion can inflame the joints and lead to changes in their alignment. The coccyx also becomes more mobile in this period and can cause problems. The coccyx is also vulnerable to damage if someone falls backwards onto a hard floor – lean people are particularly at risk from this kind of injury.

SPINAL CURVES

Although the spinal vertebrae stand one on top of each other, the column they make is not straight. Rather, the spine forms an 'S' curve. There are two inward curves in the lower back and neck, while the thoracic spine curves gently outwards. The inner curves are called the *lumbar lordosis* and *cervical lordosis*, the outward curve the *thoracic*

> **Definition**
> An inward (posteriorly concave) curve to the spine is called a lordosis, an outward (posteriorly convex) curve a kyphosis.

kyphosis. These curves are not present at birth, but begin to develop in early childhood.

In the early years of life, a baby's spine is rounded, and we call this rounded shape the 'primary spinal curve'. As the baby starts to lie on its front and lift its head up, the neck curve starts to form. It is not until a baby stands up that the curve in the lower back is formed. Because the neck and lower back curves form later, they are called 'secondary spinal curves' (see fig. 1.5).

If your spine was completely straight, a large amount of shock would be transmitted up to your head whenever you ran or jumped. The function of the spinal curves is to enable the spine to act in a spring-like fashion, absorbing some of the shock of movement.

When the spinal curves are altered, stress can be placed on the spine. This can occur through

> ## Key point
> Maintaining a correct curve in the lower back is important to overall spinal health.

alterations in posture and the way we work: long periods spent sitting at desks and driving a car will change the important curve in the lumbar region, and this can be a source of low back pain.

Another way that spinal curves can change is through exercise. Training one side of the body excessively can lead to an alteration in muscle balance (i.e. where one muscle is stronger or tighter on one side than the other), pulling the spine out of alignment. This is why a balanced exercise programme is so important. The good news, however, is that the spinal curves can often be helped using exercise therapy.

SPINAL LIGAMENTS

The spine has numerous ligaments (see fig. 1.6), which broadly fall into two categories. There are those running the length of the spine such as the *supraspinous ligament* (running over the top of the spinous processes) and the *interspinous ligament* (running between the spinous processes). Then there are ligaments associated with individual joints, such as the *ligamentum flavum*, which attaches to the facet joint. The *intertransverse ligament* attaches between the transverse processes. The *anterior longitudinal ligament* is placed at the front of the vertebral body while the *posterior longitudinal ligament* is at the back, forming the anterior wall of the spinal canal. These ligaments will limit flexion, extension and side flexion as they are placed under tension.

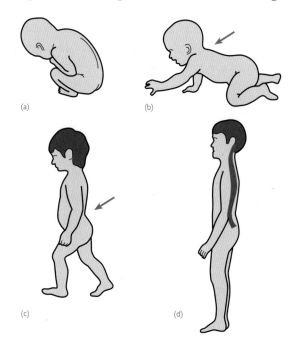

(a)   (b)

(c)   (d)

Figure 1.5 Primary and secondary spinal curves

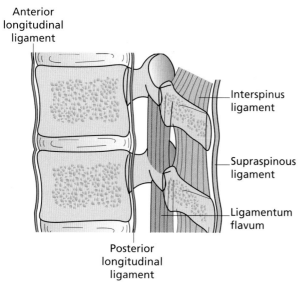

Figure 1.6 Ligaments of the spine

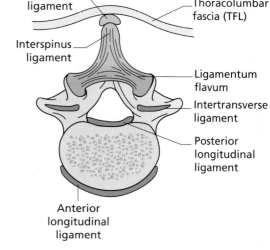

Figure 1.7 Ligamentous complex of the back

Although described separately the ligaments merge into each other. The *supraspinous ligament* merges with the *thorocolumbar fascia* and so tension from the deep abdominal muscles is transmitted through the *thorocolumbar fascia* into the *supraspinous ligament* and then directly to the vertebra. The *interspinous ligament* merges with the *supraspinous ligament* – if the two ligaments are separated, their tensile stiffness (essentially their strength) is reduced by 40 per cent. The *ligamentum flavum* merges with the joint capsule, and so is directly effected by movement of the facet joints. The combination of the supraspinous, interspinous, ligamentum flavum and thorocolumbar fascia forms a strong ligamentous complex at the back of the spine which supports the structures and transmits force. This provides one of the major stabilising mechanisms of the spine (see fig. 1.7).

Bending forwards will stretch the ligaments behind the spine while relaxing those in front. Bending backwards will reverse the situation, stretching the front ligaments while relaxing those covering the back of the spine. Side bending and rotating motions will tense ligaments on one side while relaxing (crimping) those on the other side.

Clinical note

If an exercise or posture persistently over-stretches a ligament, the ligament will inflame and become painful. This may take time to develop, so pain is not felt immediately, and backache occurs the following day. Where an individual has pain of this type it is important to analyse the movements they are using to remove the cause of the pain.

NERVES

The spinal cord consists of thousands of tiny nerve fibres bunched together much like a telephone cable. In the same way as the telephone line, the nerves carry electrical messages. When you want to move your leg, for example, an electrical message is sent from the brain. It travels down a nerve contained in your spinal cord to the muscles in your leg, commanding them to move. This is called a motor function.

A similar message can move in the opposite direction. If you touch a hot object, an electrical message is sent from your hand up a nerve in your arm through the spinal cord and to the area of your brain responsible for feeling, a process called sensory function. A third important function, which is generally less well-known, is the autonomic function. This controls the condition of the internal body environment, including blood flow to the internal organs, and condition of the skin. Changes to the autonomic function of a nerve can cause alterations such as changes in sweating (*sudomotor* effect), blood flow (*vasomotor* effect), hair response (*pilomotor* effect) and general skin condition.

At any time, thousands of electrical impulses are travelling up and down the nerves in your body. If something blocks these impulses, the electrical messages change, and both movement (motor function) and feeling (sensory function) can be affected. With longer term conditions the skin appearance can actually change (autonomic function). When you trap a nerve it is compressed, a little like stepping on a hosepipe. The impulses for movement and feeling can become blocked, you will feel tingling sensations and numbness, and your muscles may twitch or become weak. These sensations can be felt wherever the nerve travels.

Often in the lower back the feelings travel into the buttock and leg and then right down to the foot. In the upper back the sensations from the neck and thoracic spine can be felt down the arm. In both cases this is an example of 'referred pain'.

Key point

Pain or 'strange feelings' in your leg could be caused by an injury to your back. A process called referred pain.

The major nerves are covered by a sheath which insulates them in a similar way to that of an electrical cable. These nerve sheaths slide and are stretched during movement. If an injury causes swelling around a nerve, the sheath may tighten, blocking free movement and causing pain or tingling as it is stretched. This process, called 'adverse neural tension' requires specific stretching exercises targeting the nerves and muscles, and is covered in chapter 2.

DISC STRUCTURE AND FUNCTION

The disc is the structure that separates the bodies of the two adjacent spinal bones. The disc acts like a shock absorber, preventing the spine from being shaken or jarred when we walk and run. Each disc has a hard outer casing (*annulus fibrosis*) which contains a softer spongy gel called the 'disc nucleus' (*nucleus palposis*) (see fig. 1.8). Importantly, this gel has no direct blood supply, but instead relies on movement for its health. As the spine moves, fluids are pressed into the disc nucleus and waste products are squeezed out,

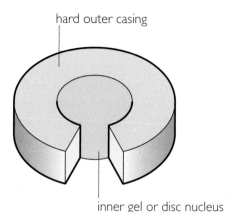

hard outer casing

inner gel or disc nucleus

Figure 1.8 Disc structure

keeping the disc healthy. As we get older the disc gel begins to dry up and becomes more brittle. When this happens the spine gets stiffer, so you are no longer able to turn the cartwheels of your youth when you retire! However, regular exercise will help the disc stay springy for longer.

If we were to look at the discs of someone who is 30 years old but inactive, and compare them to someone who is 40 but fit, the two discs would probably be exactly the same. The discs of the fitter person have stayed 'younger' because they have been subjected to regular movement.

> **Key point**
>
> The disc needs regular movement to stay healthy.

Throughout the day bodyweight compresses the disc and slowly presses water out of it. This compression causes the disc to shrink slightly and reduces its height. Although this variation is slight,

because it occurs throughout the lower spine, the overall effect is a loss of about 1 cm in body height between the morning and evenings. Exercises that involve compression, either through weight bearing (weight training) or impact (running), also cause the spinal disc to shrink. The loads taken by the spine are magnified through a process of leverage, so a moderate squat exercise can cause compression forces on the L3 and L4 discs of 6–10 times bodyweight. Research has shown that a simple 25-minute weight training session can compress the spine by 5 mm and a 6 km run by 3 mm. Constant loading with an overhead weight (such as that required by bodybuilding) can shrink the spine by over 10 mm. These changes in the lumbar discs make lumbar compression exercises unsuitable for those who have had recent spine problems such as slipped (prolapsed) discs.

> **Key point**
>
> Exercise involving high-compression loads imposed on the spine are unsuitable for a person who is recovering from a disc injury.

THE IMPORTANCE OF SPINAL FACET JOINTS

The 'facets' are two small joints at the back of the vertebrae. Their name comes from the fact that they have flat faces, and the direction in which these are orientated dictates which movements are possible in the various spinal regions. In the cervical region the facets are quite round and face upwards. The thoracic facets are more or less triangular and face backwards. The lumbar facets face upwards and inwards and are larger and stronger than the others. The direction of the facet joints means that very little rotation actually occurs in the lumbar region, rotation occurring mostly in the thoracic spine.

The facet joints are similar in construction to other synovial joints in the body in that they are contained within a tough leathery bag called a 'capsule', which merges with the outer (lateral) portion of the ligamentum flavum. As we bend forwards, the facet joint opens up, and as we bend back the joint closes. Twisting the spine results in the surfaces of the facet joint sliding over each other (see fig. 1.9).

Because these joints are so small, rapid movements can cause them to move too far, thus damaging them. Bending forwards repeatedly when practising stretching exercises, for example, can overstretch the leathery capsule of the facet joints, leaving the spine looser than it should be and therefore susceptible to injury. Bending backwards suddenly, as can be seen in some weight training exercises, closes the facet joints rapidly with a sudden 'jolt'. Over time this can cause premature wearing of these delicate joints.

> **Key point**
> Rapid movements can jolt the small facet joints at the back of the spine over and over again, causing pain and swelling.

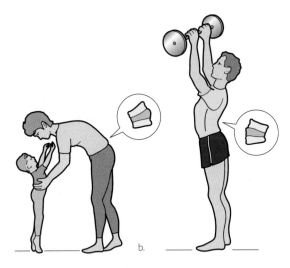

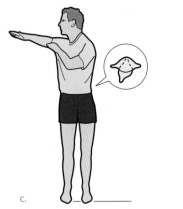

Figure 1.9 Movement of the spinal joints

SPINAL MOVEMENTS

The total extent of movement possible at any joint is called its 'range of movement'. Normally, in everyday living, we operate with our joints moving in the middle of this range. This is really the safest area of movement because the joint is in no danger of being overstretched and the muscles feel comfortable.

With each movement, damage can only occur if the joint is pressed as far as it can go. We call this end point of movement the 'end range'. When we are exercising, if we push our joints to the end range over and over again we can damage them. A safer method is to practise exercises for which the great majority of movements are in the middle of

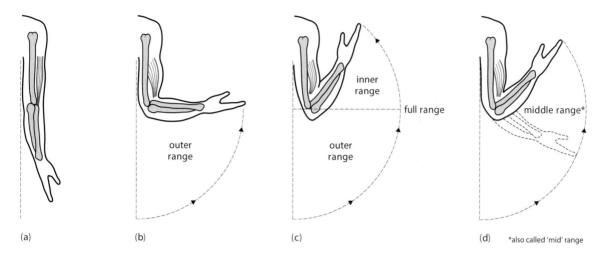

Labels within figure:
(a) outer range
(b) outer range
(c) inner range / full range / outer range
(d) middle range* / *also called 'mid' range

Figure 1.10 Range of motion

the movement range. This provides a good margin of safety (see fig. 1.10).

Gym users tend to talk about spine movements as a whole, often bending and straightening without realising that segments of the spine can move relative to each other. Instructors, however, will look at specific segments of motion, for example during an overhead shoulder exercise the thoracic spine may be flattening while the lumbar spine curves excessively. Therapists will look in even closer detail: at the individual spinal segments. For example, they are interested in the motion between L5/L4 relative to that of L4/L3. Motion of an individual spinal segment can be impor-

tant because stiffness in one segment following injury may cause a neighbouring segment to move excessively (this is called 'compensatory hypermobility') causing pain. The answer to this is to make the stiff segment move more so that the lax segment can move less. A physiotherapist will often use joint manipulation to release a stiff spinal segment, followed by exercise therapy to re-educate the muscles supporting the lax segment.

When we get to end range in a movement, what are the factors that limit us? During forward bending (flexion), the anterior portion of the disc is compressed while the posterior portion is placed under tension. The total volume of the disc remains unchanged and so theoretically should discal pressure (the pressure within the soft nucleus at the centre of the disc). However, tension in the soft tissues causes an alteration in disc or pressure. If we look at one of the centre lumbar discs (L3) and record its pressure in standing at 100 per cent, lying the discal pressure reduces to just 25 per cent. Bending movements, however, increase discal pressure. Bending forwards gives a pressure recording of 150 per cent and this is dramatically increased to 220 per cent when lifting a small (10 kg) weight. These changes in pressure are important during rehabilitation if somebody has a history of disc injury. It is vital to choose a starting position with low discal pressure, such as lying with the knees flexed. The range of motion to lumbar flexion is to a large part determined by the height of the lumbar discs. In a young (especially female) person the disc height is at its maximum so the range of motion is greatest. Disc height, and with it the range of lumbar flexion, can reduce with ageing. As the lumbar vertebrae tilt into flexion, posteriorly placed facet joints are opened and the facet joint capsules, together with the posteriorly placed ligaments, are stretched. In dissection experiments, the disc has been shown to limit range of motion to flexion by 29 per cent, the *supraspinatus* and *intraspinatus* ligaments by 19 per cent and facet joint capsules by nearly 40 per cent. In the forward bending posture with the body angled at the hip, shearing stress is caused to the facet joints of the lumbar spine as the top vertebra slides forward. The combination of alteration in discal pressure, stretching and shearing forces makes repeated flexion of the lumbar spine potentially dangerous.

As we will see later (chapter 3) reducing the total amount of forward bending a client performs is a fundamental principle of good back care.

> **Definition**
> Shearing forces are those that push one part of the body in one direction, and another part of the body in the opposite direction.

When assessing a person's range of motion with regard to flexion it is important to pay attention to three areas. Firstly determine the amount of anterior pelvic tilt compared to the amount of lumbar motion. Anterior pelvic tilt may be assessed by the vertical movement of the front of the pelvis (anterior superior iliac spine), a large vertical movement indicating greater anterior tilt. Lumbar motion can be observed as a total amount (range) seen by the depth of the lumbar curve, a deeper curve showing greater movement. Individual movements between each vertebral bone may be assessed by feeling (palpating) movement of the spinous processes relative to each other.

Secondly, observe the curvature of the lumbar spine. In standing the normal curvature (lordosis) should be present. Flattening of the lumbar lordosis indicates the beginning of flexion of the lumbar spine. In this situation the tissue stress described above will be present. In positions such as slumped sitting, for example, the lumbar spine can be flexed to a point where its lordosis is obliterated (i.e. it no longer curves as it should). This postural setup is a common cause of overuse symptoms to the lower back. The movement cycle of the lumbar spine is: lordosis, flattening of lordosis and, finally, lumbar flexion.

During lumbar extension the situation is reversed. Now the anterior structures are placed under tension while the posterior structures are initially relaxed, then compressed. The anterior portion of the spinal disc is placed under tension to keep the portion compressed. The facet joints close and the joint surfaces impact. Further extension stress on the lumbar spine causes the vertebra to pivot around the axis formed by decompressing facet joints. Extension therefore causes traction to the lumbar disc. Both rotation and lateral flexion movements cause twisting of the disc and opening of the facet joints on one side and closing on the other. The orientation of the facet joints within the lumbar spine means that only a small range of rotation is available (approximately 5°).

The thick cartilage covering of the flat facet joint surface causes an anatomical cushion during rotation with 0.5 mm of compression for every 1° of rotation. As the disc is stretched and placed under traction it provides 35 per cent of the total resistance to rotation.

LUMBAR AND PELVIC MOVEMENTS

Excessive movement in the lumbar spine can occur without us noticing it. If a person bends forwards to touch their toes or backwards to look at the ceiling, the movement is obvious. But there is another – more subtle – way in which the lumbar spine can move.

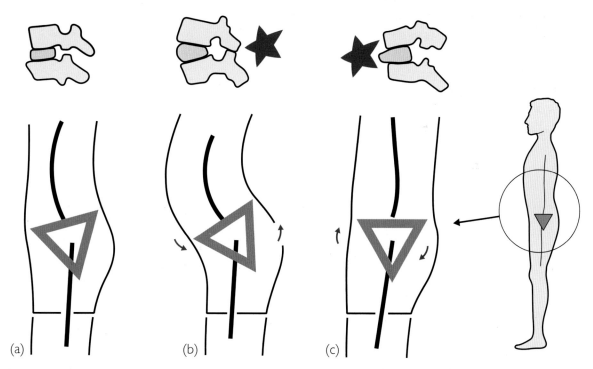

Figure 1.11 Pelvic movement (a. neutral position, b. anterior tilt, c. posterior tilt)

The pelvis is connected directly to the lumbar spine (see fig. 1.11), and in turn balances on the hip joints rather like a seesaw. Because it is balanced, the pelvis can tilt forwards and backwards. As it tilts, the pelvis pulls the spine with it. If the pelvis tips down, the arch in the lumbar spine increases in a way that is equivalent to moving the spine backwards into 'extension'. When the pelvis tilts up the lumbar curve is flattened, and the movement in the lumbar spine is equivalent to flexion, or forward bending.

If the movement of the pelvis is excessive, the spine is in turn pulled to its end range, placing stress on the spinal tissues. Note that it is only the lumbar spine that is moving. The rest of the spine remains largely unchanged, so the person is still standing upright.

The ratio between movement of the lumbar spine on the pelvis and movement of the pelvis on the hip joints is important, and this combined motion of the two segments is called the lumbo-pelvic rhythm. For example, when you bend forwards to reach down to a desk from a standing position, you have a choice. You could lock your pelvis and bend only from the spine, secondly you could keep your spine stiff and move from your hip alone or thirdly you could combine the two movements and move from both your hips and spine. The third motion is actually the one that places the least stress on the body. By moving the pelvis on the hips, the requirement for spine bending (lumbar flexion) is reduced so the lumbar discs are protected. If, however, you keep your spine completely rigid, the lumbar muscles are overworked and can go into spasm and cause muscle pain. Ideally, you should use twice as much pelvic movement as lumbar movement in everyday activities (a lumbo-pelvic ratio of 1:2). Commonly, however, people often forget to move from their pelvis and so the lumbar spine does most of the work, giving a lumbo-pelvic ratio of 3:1 with the pelvis moving only when the lumbar spine has moved to its end range.

> ## Key point
>
> When bending forwards the ratio of lumbar movement (flexion) to pelvic movement (anterior tilt) is called the lumbo-pelvic rhythm. Ideally this should be 1:2 when bending for objects at table height.

The range of anterior pelvic tilt is to a large extent dictated by the tightness of the hamstring muscles. The hamstrings are attached to the *ischial tuberosity* (also known as the 'sitting bones' at the sides of the inner pelvis) and as a result tightness will anchor the tuberosity and prevent anterior pelvic tilt. This situation is made worse in cases where the knees are locked, pre-stretching the lower part of the hamstrings. In an individual with tight hamstrings forward bending with the knee locked will often cause flexion to be imposed on the lumbar spine without any significant anterior pelvic tilt. To reduce the range of lumbar flexion it is necessary to slightly flex (or unlock) then release hamstring tension and allow anterior pelvic tilt, causing the upper portion of the hamstrings to stretch as the ischial tuberosity moves upwards.

> ## Key point
>
> Movement of the pelvis directly affects the lumbar spine.

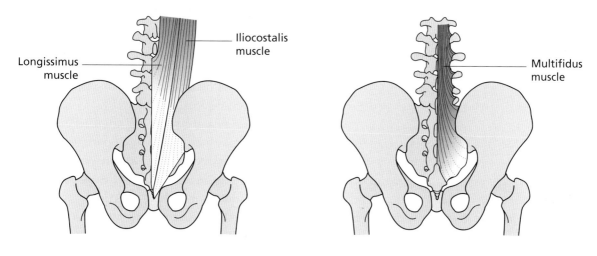

Longissimus muscle

Iliocostalis muscle

Multifidus muscle

Figure 1.12 Major muscles of the lower trunk

MUSCLES OF THE LOWER TRUNK

We need to become familiar with all of the muscles affecting the lower trunk, that is the area between the ribcage (above) and the pelvic bones (below). At the front and sides of the trunk are the four principal abdominal muscles, at the back the spinal muscles and at the base of the trunk and actually within the pelvic bones themselves the pelvic floor muscles. We are also concerned with the hip muscles, because as we have seen hip, pelvic and lumbar motion are intimately linked (see fig 1.12).

ABDOMINAL MUSCLES

In the centre of the abdomen is the *rectus abdominis*. This muscle runs from the lower ribs to the pubic region, forming a narrow strap. It tapers down from about 15 cm (6 in) wide at the top to 8 cm (3 in) wide at the bottom. The muscle has three fibrous bands across it at the

level of the navel, and above and below this point (see fig. 1.12). The rectus muscle on each side of the body is contained within a sheath, the two sheaths merging in the centre line of the body via a strong fibrous band called the *linea alba*. This region splits during pregnancy to allow for the bulk of the developing child (see chapter 3).

At the side of the abdomen there are two diagonal muscles, the internal oblique and the external oblique (see fig. 1.13). The internal oblique attaches to the front of the pelvic bone and a strong ligament in this region. From here it travels up and across to the lower ribs and into the sheath covering the rectus muscle. The external oblique has a similar position, but lies at an angle to the internal oblique. The external oblique begins from the lower eight ribs and travels to the sheath covering the rectus muscle and to the strong pelvic ligaments. The fibres in the centre of the muscle travel diagonally, but those on the edge travel vertically and will assist the rectus muscle in its action.

Underneath the oblique abdominals lies the *transversus abdominis*. This attaches from the pelvic bones and tissue covering the spinal muscles and travels forward horizontally to merge with the sheath covering the rectus muscle. Figure 1.13 shows a cross-section of the trunk. In the centre you can see the rectus muscle surrounded by connective tissue called the 'rectus sheath'. This sheath of the two neighbouring muscles joins in the centre to form the *linea alba*. At the side of the trunk you can see the three distinct layers of muscles, from the inside out-transversus, internal oblique and external oblique.

At the side and back of the trunk, the *quadratus lumborum* muscle is also important (see fig. 1.13). It is positioned between the pelvis and rib cage, and has an inner and outer portion. The inner portion is attached directly to the spine and is therefore an important muscle in stability. The outer portion has a tendency to get tight and painful during back pain.

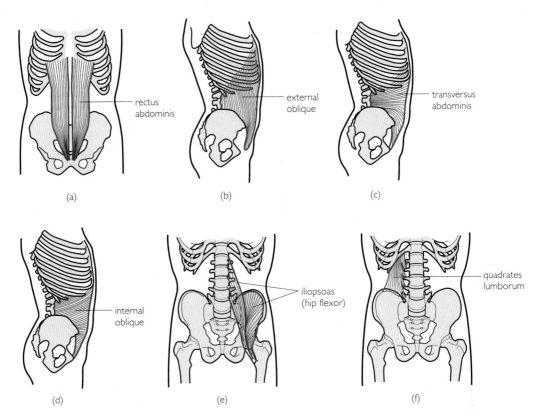

(a) rectus abdominis
(b) external oblique
(c) transversus abdominis
(d) internal oblique
(e) iliopsoas (hip flexor)
(f) quadrates lumborum

Figure 1.13 Cross-section of the trunk

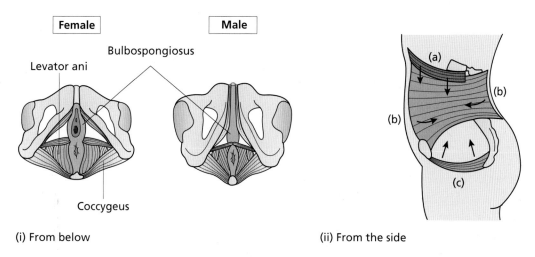

Female **Male**

Bulbospongiosus

Levator ani

Coccygeus

(i) From below

(a)

(b)

(b)

(c)

(ii) From the side

Figure 1.14 Pelvic floor muscles. RH figure from the side in relation to the abdominal wall. (a) Diaphragm, (b) Oblique abdominals, (c) Pelvic floor

PELVIC FLOOR MUSCLES

When performing abdominal exercises to enhance core stability you must also be aware of the pelvic floor muscles. These attach to the inside of the pelvis and form a sort of sling running from the tailbone (coccyx) at the back to the pubic bone (crotch) at the front.

The pelvic floor group consists of the *levator ani*, *coccygeus*, and *bulbospongiosus* (see fig. 1.14). The levator ani form a floor for the base of the pelvis, attaching to the inner surface of the pubis and pelvis and joining together centrally. This midline portion of the muscles is separated to form the urethra, anus and, in the female, the vagina. These openings are controlled by rings of muscle called *sphincters* which lie in the pelvic floor. The coccygeus is a flat triangular muscle attaching the back of the pelvis (*ischium*) to the coccyx. As well as its function with levator ani in pelvic floor support, the coccygeus is able to move the coccyx (during childbirth and going to the toilet). The

bulbospongiosus is responsible for erection (penis in the male, clitoris in the female). It also closes the vagina and is active during orgasm in both sexes. The pelvic floor muscles are important for both men and women. They are essential for core stability following back pain and may be damaged during pregnancy or prostate surgery; re-education of these muscles is vital in both sexes.

Key point

The pelvic floor muscles are important in both men and women. Muscle re-education is vital after childbirth and various forms of surgery.

BACK EXTENSOR MUSCLES

There are two groups of back extensor muscles which are important to core stability, especially in lifting. The first are local muscles that attach between each of the vertebrae covering a single spinal segment. The second are global muscles, which attach along the whole length of the spine, spanning several spinal segments (see also chapter 4).

Of the local group, the *multifidus* muscle is particularly important. This not only moves the spinal bones in relation to each other – in other words, it produces a rocking action of one bone against the other – but also flattens the lumbar curve without moving the whole spine. Probably the most important feature of this muscle, however, is its ability to stiffen the spine. Because it is positioned between the spinal bones, it acts a little like cement between bricks. A column of bricks stacked on top of each other is very unstable. However, if the bricks are cemented together with mortar, they are very stable. Any amount of pressing and pulling will be withstood, and the column will remain standing. The multifidus has a similar function in that it stiffens the spine and helps it to resist bending forces. However, after a back injury or bout of low back pain, it becomes much smaller and weaker leaving the spine more susceptible to further injury. Unfortunately, even after the back pain has been resolved, the multifidus does not build itself back up again readily. It needs to be 'reminded' how to work through the use of a specialist form of training known as *sensorimotor retraining* (see chapter 4).

The global spinal muscles are the spinal extensors, which lie on either side of the spine. These consist of several muscles, the two most important being a central muscle (*longissimus*) which travels close to the spine and a more side placed muscle (*iliocostalis*) which attaches to the ribs (see fig. 1.12, p. 15). Together, they are like two powerful columns that support the spine as we bend forwards and move the back from a vertical to a more horizontal position. Although the strength of these muscles is important, their endurance – how long they can hold themselves tight – is actually more significant. This is because if the endurance of the muscles is poor, they will gradually allow the back to slip into an increasingly poor posture after repeated bending activities.

Think of the spine as a fishing rod, if the rod has weakened over time any fish caught on the line will cause the rod to bend, not just big ones! The result is the same with regard to weight placed on the back. The rod, or in this case the spine, bends more and more. Therefore the amount of time someone can spend tightening the back muscles and holding them tight is the important factor, especially with intensive activities such as sport or heavy lifting. This is why we target these muscles with a number of exercises, ultimately leading to the leg extension over bench shown on page 137. The way that you lift an object and the function of your spine as a lever during your lifting posture is covered in chapter 8.

THE HIP MUSCLES

The major hip muscle affected during abdominal training is the hip flexor (*iliopsoas*). This muscle is made up of two parts, the first coming from the lumbar spine (*psoas*), the second from the pelvis (*iliacus*) (see fig. 1.13e). Both parts merge to fasten on to the top of the thighbone (*femur*). The action of this muscle is best illustrated when lying flat on your back. If you lift one leg, the hip flexor has acted to bend the hip. If you sit up from lying flat, keeping your back straight and bending at the hip joint, the muscle has acted to pull your trunk up.

Because the psoas muscle attaches to each vertebra of the lumbar spine, as it contracts it pulls the lumbar vertebrae together. As this happens the pressure within the vertebra will increase. This has two effects, one good and one bad. Slight pressure will help to hold the vertebra in place, thereby stabilising them. As pressure increases further, however, the spinal discs can distort causing them to press closer to the nerves in the area causing pain. This effect is made greater when the spine is not optimally aligned – too bent or too hollow. Minimising (but not obliterating) work of the iliopsoas during abdominal training and ensuring that the lower back is in its neutral position when the iliopsoas is working is a key feature of good abdominal exercise practice in general, but is particularly important for beginners.

Key point

If the iliopsoas muscle is worked too hard it can pull excessively on the lower spine, dangerously increasing the pressure within the discs.

MUSCLE ACTION

The trunk muscles often work together (in synergistic action), and so in any movement involving the abdomen, most of the muscles will be active to a certain extent at some point in the movement range. In a sit-up action, the iliopsoas works and the upper portion of the rectus is emphasised. In pelvic tilting the lower portion of the rectus and the outer fibres of the external oblique are used. Twisting actions involve the oblique abdominals, while the transversus acting with the obliques pulls the stomach in tight. This muscle is also used in coughing and sneezing. Together with the obliques, the outer portion of the quadratus is important for side bending actions and also pulls on the lower ribs when breathing deeply. The inner portion is next to the spine and helps to support it in actions that tend to pull the body sideways. The quadratus is therefore important to core stability when carrying an object in one hand – for example, a shopping basket or suitcase. After pregnancy, certain types of lower back pain, some types of surgery and in very obese individuals, the pelvic floor muscles reduce their tone and people can sometimes lose control of the sphincters and dribble urine. For this reason, regaining control of the pelvic floor is important and can be achieved at the same time as re-educating the deep muscle corset (transversus and internal oblique). As we shall see in chapter 4, the pelvic floor muscles are also integral to the creation of pressure, which forms the 'abdominal balloon', an important process in developing core stability.

The abdominal muscles can be used for movement – to bend or twist the trunk, for example – or for stability. When used for stability, the muscles hold the spine firm, preventing excessive movement. In order to do this, they work to make the trunk into a more solid cylinder. For instance, when we are lifting something or pushing and pulling, the spine has to form a solid base for the arms and legs to push against. If not, the force created by the limbs will move the trunk rather than the object. The mechanisms of spinal stabilisation are covered in chapter 4.

THE NEUTRAL POSITION OF THE LUMBAR SPINE

We have seen that as we move the spine the alignment of the spinal bones and tissues changes. For example, as we flex forwards the facet joints open and the tissues on the back of the spine stretch, while those on the front relax. At the same time the pressure within the spinal discs increases. This combination of pressure and stretch, if repeated over and over again, can damage the spinal tissues.

If, however, we align the spinal tissues so the spine is upright and the lumbar region is comfortably curved, the spinal tissues are now at their normal length and the pressure within the discs is lowered. We call this normal alignment of the spine the 'neutral position' (see fig. 1.15). It is one of the safest postures for the spine, so all the foundation movements that we use begin with the spine in its neutral position.

To find your own neutral position, stand with your back to a wall. Your buttocks and shoulders should touch the wall. Place the flat of your hand between the wall and the small of your back. Try to tilt your pelvis so you flatten your back and then tilt your pelvis the other way so you increase the hollow in the lower back. Your neutral position (which will be slightly different for each person) is halfway between the flat and the hollow positions.

> **Key point**
> In the neutral position the spine is correctly aligned and the spinal tissues are held at the right length.

> **Key point**
> Use of tactile cueing with a partner can help them find neutral position of the lumbar spine.

You should only just be able to place the flat of your hand between your back and the wall. If you can only place your fingers through, your back is too flat; if your whole hand up to your wrist can pass through the space, your back is too hollow.

To find neutral position on a client or training partner, have them stand up against a wall with their hands out in front with arms straight (standing press up position). Stand behind them side on, and – with their permission – reach your

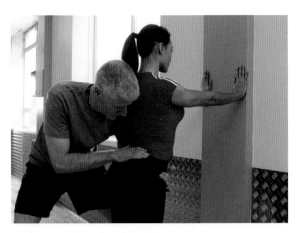

Figure 1.15 Finding another person's neutral lumbar spine position

left forearm around their waist placing it across their waistband. Press your left shoulder against the back of their ribcage and the flat of your right hand over their sacrum (i.e. the rear of the pelvis). Their upper body is effectively fixed by their hands on the wall (they must keep their arms straight) and your left shoulder pressing against the back of their ribcage. Your left hand monitors the front of their pelvis and your right the back. Using this position you can help them to tilt their pelvis using your hands to guide or 'cue' the movement. Using touch in this fashion to give feedback is called tactile cueing and is an effective way of teaching, often cutting down many frustrating hours of practice for a client. Initially simply tilt the pelvis trying to encourage full range of movement, and then stop in the neutral position.

Finding the neutral position of the lumbar spine involves precision movements of the pelvis and lumbar spine combined with alteration in muscle tension around the hips. This combination demands good *proprioception* and this can be enhanced in several ways. One method is to encourage clients to reproduce a movement either passively or actively. For passive reproduction of movement, the therapist or personal trainer tilts the client's pelvis and asks them to identify the neutral position. This can be useful in situations where the client is unable to perform a pelvic tilt action at will. Active reproduction of movement comes later, and this involves the client performing pelvic tilt actions within a predetermined motion range. Both of these actions can be performed in the clinic and once perfected can be repeated in a group exercise situation. Clinical Pilates is often the exercise of choice for this movement, as pelvic tilting is one of the foundation (or 'baseline') movements and will be included in many classes.

Definition

Proprioception is the awareness of both the relative positions of different parts of the body and the effort the body expends in moving.

// BACK CONDITIONS

2

It is important to have an appreciation of the types of medical conditions (*pathologies*) from which your clients may suffer. It is the responsibility of the medical practitioner or qualified therapist to make an accurate diagnosis, but equally it is the responsibility of the personal trainer to be aware of tissue condition as a result of pathology. Although a diagnosis is important to rule out potentially serious medical conditions, in some cases it can impair progress of rehabilitation. People may often think that there is little point in participating in a rehabilitation programme if they have been told that a medical condition will not progress. For example, where someone has arthritic changes in the spine they may have been shown an x-ray and told that these changes are permanent. Some individuals with such changes may have full function of the spine, while others (even those with fewer relevant changes) may have gross impairment. Full function depends on an interaction between all of the tissues, as well as physical and mental factors. As we will see later, fear of movement can often be more limiting than tissue pathology, and fear of movement can be increased by a diagnosis given without sufficient explanation. Rehabilitation targets not only the tissues but the mind, giving confidence

and enabling the client to see progress. In my 35 years as a physiotherapist many treatments have come and gone but the one consistent feature is the importance of exercise therapy. It is a serious mistake to underestimate the power of this technique even where the medical outlook may seem poor. The human body is trained through movement, and correctly prescribed exercise therapy should be a part of most treatments when targeting the spine.

DISC INJURY

We have seen in chapter 1 that pressure within the spinal discs changes both with movement and throughout the day. As the spinal vertebrae move relative to each other, tension changes within soft tissues cause alterations within the nucleus of the disc. In addition, throughout the day the water content of the nucleus reduces and spinal shrinkage occurs over time. The central nucleus is contained within the outer shell of the disc (*annulus fibrosis*). During flexion the nucleus of the disc is pressed backwards in the opposite direction to the imposed force. The analogy here is of a toothpaste tube, where squeezing the base of the tube causes the toothpaste to move in the opposite direction towards the open end of the tube. In the case of the spine the nuclear material within the disc centre is moving closer to the nerves positioned at the back of the spine. The combination of increased pressure and degeneration of the vertebral casing can cause small cracks in the casing itself. Initially the change in the disc through repeated flexion stress is one of alteration of the disc's shape. Over time part of the nuclear material within the disc centre can work its way through small hairline cracks within the disc casing. Eventually disc material can appear on the outer edge of the disc, forming what is colloquially termed a slipped disc or more accurately a disc prolapse. The bulge moves backwards and is forced slightly to one side by the posterior spinal ligaments, which are positioned centrally. The nuclear material from the disc presses against the delicate root of the nerve causing alteration in both sensory and motor impulses.

Definition

A prolapsed (or slipped) disc is the movement of some of the gel-like centre of the disc through the disc casing. Once through, the gel may press on a nerve causing pain.

It is important to note that the blood flow to discs is very poor, and where the nuclear material has moved outside the disc annulus it no longer has access to nutrients from the blood. Almost immediately the disc bulge (prolapse) will begin to dry and shrink away from the compressed nerve root. Contact with the nerve will however cause local swelling and nerve irritation, the effects of which will last after the prolapsed material has dried and shrunk away. Pain from the injury and the alteration in both sensory and motor impulses causes local muscle changes. Firstly, nervous impulses are unable to travel normally and so the number of nerve impulses is reduced leading to *poor recruitment* of local muscles. In addition the body tries to protect itself from further injury by instigating a process of *inhibition*. This means that other nerve impulses are generated which deliberately prevent movement by reducing tone in the muscles surrounding the injured area.

Definition

Poor recruitment occurs when fewer nerve impulses reach a muscle. Inhibition occurs when a second nerve tries to stop the muscle from working.

The combination of enforced rest, pain and local muscle inhibition causes debilitating changes to the damaged area. The primary injury is one of movement of discal material. However, the secondary injury – brought on by the local muscle response – will remain long after the primary injury has been resolved. The aim of rehabilitation is to protect the spine from further injury during the primary stage and slowly redevelop movement in the secondary stage.

As we will see, when we look at the principles of rehabilitation in chapter 4, enhancing the stability mechanisms of the lumbar spine can greatly reduce pressure within the discs and consequently may reduce the possibility of discal damage.

BACK PAIN IN OBESITY

Unfortunately we live at the beginning of an obesity epidemic. This has effects on low back pain in two principal ways. Firstly, the increased weight of an obese individual causes high levels of compression within the lumbar spine. Compression increases intradiscal pressure within the nucleus of the lower lumbar vertebrae in particular. Over time this causes a reduction in discal height with pronounced discal bulging. Secondly, compression causes increased loading of the facet joints. In the short term this can cause local inflammatory responses but in the long term joint erosion is more likely. The local changes to the lumbar spine which occur as a result of obesity are paralleled by postural changes to this body area. As we have seen the pelvis pivots on the hip joint much like a seesaw, with the abdominal muscles and spinal extensors pulling upwards and the hip flexors and hip extensors pulling down. Obesity also sees an increase in local body fat (central obesity) and often a reduction in tone to the abdominal muscles.

Definition

Central obesity (also known as abdominal obesity) is the accumulation of fat around the abdomen. The fat is laid down beneath the skin (subcutaneous fat) and around the internal organs (visceral fat).

The increased weight of abdominal fat pulls downwards, lengthening the superficial abdominal muscles. The reduction in support provided by the muscles allows the viscera to move forwards of the body posture line, effectively making the internal organs heavier. This leverage change causes the internal organs to move forwards and downwards and the abdominal wall to lengthen in its lower part (*visceral ptosis*). The result is a protruding abdominal wall, which seems to hang in folds from the inguinal ligament. Now the seesaw effect of the pelvis is disrupted, allowing the pelvis to anteriorly tilt and shorten the hip flexor muscles. The hip extensor muscles are lengthened and lose tone while the spinal extensor muscles become firm and tight. Increased anterior pelvic tilt causes a deepening of the lumbar lordosis and impaction of the lumbar facet joints. The gluteal muscles waste to create a classic 'pelvic crossed syndrome'. Obesity often goes hand-in-hand with low levels of physical activity, especially in young adolescents. A recent study (Shiri *et al*, 2013) showed the rate of low back pain to be 1.7 times greater in obese individuals compared to normal subjects. Interestingly, in overweight individuals, the incidence of low back pain is greater only in those who are physically inactive, so it seems that physical activity gives some protection against the development of low back pain. The development of obesity during adolescence can be used as a predictor of low back pain in later life, especially in females. Encouraging school-age children to become active and providing weight management consultation is a vital element of preventive health care for this condition.

Managing low back pain in obese individuals involves a combination of dietary advice, general activity increase, and postural re-education. While activity is important, early movement when the low back is in an irritable state is unwise. Pain should be targeted first, with a progressive increase in physical activity being encouraged as pain subsides. Once activity levels increase it

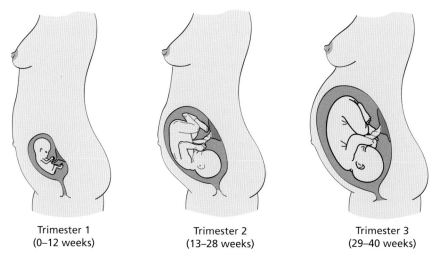

Trimester 1
(0–12 weeks)

Trimester 2
(13–28 weeks)

Trimester 3
(29–40 weeks)

Figure 2.1 Postural changes throughout pregnancy

becomes easier for the individual to lose weight, and at this stage dietary advice becomes vital.

Postural correction exercises can be built in to an exercise programme once lumbar pain has resolved. The aim is for a reduction in the increased depth of the lumbar lordosis to attain the lordotic posture described in chapter 3. Shortening the abdominal muscles, tightening the gluteals and releasing tightness in the spinal extensors are all important, as is re-education of the correct neutral position of the lumbar spine. Exercises such as flattening the back against a wall combine several elements of lumbar postural correction at the same time, and so generally give good client compliance.

BACK PAIN AND PREGNANCY

Pregnancy typically lasts for 40 weeks and is divided into 14-week phases called trimesters. In the first trimester the mother feels very tired and often experiences morning sickness and heartburn. Postural changes are gradual, and any back pain which occurs is likely the result of hormonal changes. The second trimester sees greater postural changes as the uterus expands, and typically mothers experience breast tenderness, and pain in the back, groin and thighs. There may also be swelling of the ankles. It is the last trimester that sees the greatest postural changes in relation to the low back, as the abdominal muscles lengthen. The developing baby 'drops' and moves lower in the abdomen, increasing the pelvic tilt and lumbar lordosis.

Definition

Pregnancy typically lasts for 40 weeks and is divided into 3 phases or trimesters, each lasting 12–14 weeks. The first trimester (weeks 0–12) is characterised by morning sickness, the second (weeks 13–28) sees the sex of the fetus becoming apparent. The third trimester (weeks 29–40) is the period of greatest weight gain.

While increases in abdominal distension during pregnancy are similar to those of obesity there are significant differences. Firstly, obesity takes some time to occur and as a consequence the abdominal muscles are lengthened over time and often weaken due to inactivity. During pregnancy, the early phases see little change to the length of the abdominal muscles and it is only within the third trimester that these changes become clinically significant. The timescale for abdominal muscle lengthening is therefore much shorter. In addition many young women remain active during pregnancy and as a consequence abdominal muscle tone is maintained. The rapid increase in the size of the developing child outpaces the ability of the abdominal muscles to lengthen. To compensate, the rectus abdominis splits in the centre (diastasis rectus abdominis) and the developing child presses through the centre of the muscle. The diastasis may increase to as much as 10 cm. In addition, in order to facilitate muscle lengthening and changes in the mobility of the pelvic joints, there are significant hormonal changes. Progesterone, oestrogen, and relaxin hormone concentrations all change. The consequence is a softening of pelvic joints with increased motion range at the sacroiliac and pubic joints. Management of back pain during pregnancy involves supporting the weight of the developing child, often using an elasticated belt which surrounds the waist and is located below the child to support some of its weight and descended position. Resting positions are chosen to reduce the lumbar lordosis and support the pelvis.

Following childbirth hormone concentrations will normalise and pelvic joint mobility will, in most cases, reduce to normal levels. In individuals where this fails to occur at the right time, specialist physiotherapy treatment is required. Two major types of intervention are normally required following pregnancy. The first is to shorten and tighten the abdominal muscles using inner range holding activities. This begins with abdominal hollowing actions to draw the abdominal wall inwards, and is followed by shortening movements for the rectus abdominis. Enhancing core stability provides increased support to the pelvic joints and in cases of pelvic pain is used in parallel with local physiotherapy management. Dietary intervention may be required where bodyweight has increased, and advice on general activity increase is warranted. In addition, the increased demands of childcare involving picking up the baby should not be overlooked. Functional training to include guidance on bending, lifting and reaching can be included within an exercise programme. Pilates exercises such as 'monkey squat' (see p. 208) can be helpful, and gym-based exercises such as light dead-lift actions can be helpful. Failure to manage low back pain following childbirth may lead to an exacerbation of the condition during a second pregnancy. Often the emphasis of healthcare is on the child with little focus on the health of the mother. Of course, the mother's health is clearly vital and gym- or exercise-based classes provide the ideal environment for this.

ADVERSE NEURAL TENSION

Adverse neural tension (ANT) can occur following injury to the disc or nerve. Nerves are made up of thousands of fibres contained within a nerve sheath. The composition can be compared to a bicycle brake cable where a sheath surrounds the cable to facilitate movement. In the case of the nerves two movements should normally occur: sliding and stretching. As we bend and straighten our limbs, our muscles contract and joints move. In order to prevent damage to the nerves, the nerves must change their length and in many cases can do so by up to 20 per cent. For example, when moving from full flexion to full extension of the spine the spinal cord can lengthen by as much as 10 cm. Most of this movement occurs in the more mobile sections of spinal cord at the neck (cervical spine) and lower back (lumbar spine). The reason for this localisation of movement is due to tension points within the nervous system. The cord is anchored (tethered) within the cervical spine (C6), thoracic spine (T6) and lumbar spine (L4). Parts of the nervous system can also move in relation to others; a process known as 'intra-neural movement'. For example the spinal cord can slide within its sheath (*dura mater*), or one nerve fibre may move in relation to the others within a nerve bundle. When performing a lateral flexion movement, the convex side of the spinal cord moves

Definition

The brain and spinal cord are surrounded by three layers of membrane called meninges. The outermost layer, closest to the surface of the body, is called the dura mater. The middle layer is the arachnoid mater and the innermost layer, closest to the brain and spinal cord is the pia mater.

to a greater degree than the concave side, the difference being as much as 15 per cent.

Following injury, nerves may be compressed and this can lead to bruising and swelling. Injuries of this type can prevent the normal tension changes within a nerve and lead to adverse nervous tension. This condition can be managed with manual therapy techniques administered by a physiotherapist to release the nerve, followed by gentle neural stretching using specific stretching exercises and localised nerve movements. To establish the presence of ANT the physiotherapist will use a number of nerve tests. In the case of the lumbar spine the two most common are the straight leg raise (SLR) and slump test. For the straight leg raise, the client lies flat on the floor or treatment couch and the leg is lifted (hip flexion) keeping the knee locked. If pain occurs it may be caused by tightness in the hamstring muscles or irritation of the sciatic nerve. Further stretch is placed on the body by pulling the toes and foot upwards (dorsiflexion) and bending (flexing) the neck. Both of these actions have no effect on the hamstring muscles and so any increase in pain must be coming from the nerve itself. For the slump test the client sits on a stool or the side of a treatment couch with their feet off the floor and their hands linked behind their back. The action is to

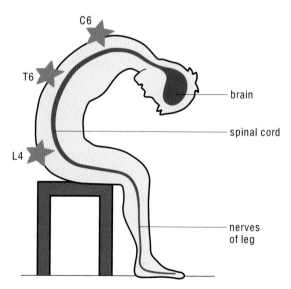

Figure 2.2 Tension points in the nervous system

flex the spine, drawing the head downwards aiming the nose towards the navel. At the same time the relevant leg is straightened and the foot dorsiflexed. When pain occurs the head is released into extension and if ANT is present pain in the leg should reduce. The slump test is used in cases of low back pain which cause referred pain in the leg, and also in cases of hamstring injury where swelling from torn muscle may actually spread to the nerve. Treatment

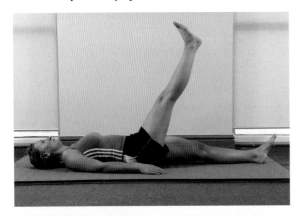

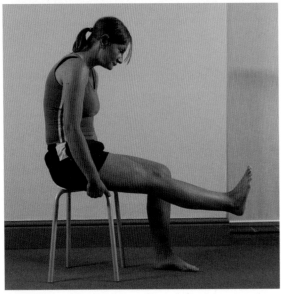

Figure 2.3 Straight leg raise and slump test

is again local to the nerve and additionally involves gentle nerve stretches. To target the sciatic nerve the two tests are simply converted into stretching exercises. The straight leg raise is performed using a belt or towel over the foot. The action should combine hip flexion with knee extension and ankle dorsiflexion. The point of maximum stretch is held for 30 to 60 seconds but at a movement range that causes only mild stretch and minimal discomfort. Nerves are easily irritated and to push further into the painful range can often aggravate the condition. The slump test is converted into a stretch by straightening the leg and dorsiflexing the foot. The position is held for 30 to 60 seconds and tension may be varied using alterations in the neck or arm position. Where pain is intense, you should choose a neutral position of the cervical spine and bring the hands forward to place them onto the subject's lap. As pain subsides initially the hands are placed behind the back and the cervical spine remains neutral, and finally the three movements, leg extension, shoulder extension (hands clasped), and cervical flexion are combined. For further details of nerve stretches, see chapter 12 in Norris (2007), *The Complete Guide to Stretching*, 3rd ed.

OSTEOPOROSIS

Osteoporosis is a condition in which bones lose minerals. Over the course of ageing normally, everyone will experience a small amount of mineral loss: on average about 3 per cent per decade. With osteoporosis this value is increased to about 10 per cent per decade and this profoundly weakens the bones. Osteoporosis may be either 'primary' (due to age) or 'secondary' (as a result of another medical condition). The most common forms of primary osteoporosis occur after the menopause (in females) or as a result of the natural ageing process (this is called senile osteoporosis, and is discussed in further detail below). The reduced mineral density (rarefaction) makes fracture of bones more likely, with the head and vertebrae being most at risk. Bone mineral density (BMD) may be assessed by x-ray or using a dual energy x-ray absorptiometry scan of the heel bone (calcaneus). Results are given in grams per centimetre squared (g/cm2), and are compared to normal values of an age matched group.

The major factors important for the development of osteoporosis are diet, oestrogen levels and physical activity. Osteoporosis is most common in obese, inactive middle-aged females. Chronic pain in the spine or hip with no evidence of injury should be investigated by the client's GP. Bone mineral loss can lead to an alteration in the normal cuboid shape of the vertebra causing anterior wedging of thoracic vertebrae. Over time the wedging increases the thoracic kyphosis giving the subject a humped appearance.

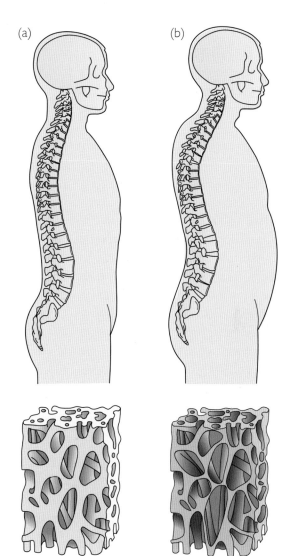

Figure 2.4 (a) Normal spinal alignment and bone density. (b) Increased thoracic curve and rarefied bone typical of Osteoporosis

Exercise therapy is used to slow the postural changes that occur in osteoporosis, and the emphasis should be on shoulder refraction and spinal extension. Activities such as sternal lift

> **Definition**
>
> Ground reaction force is the force exerted by the ground in opposition the force the body exerts on it – if a body is pushing forwards and down, the ground reaction force will be back and up.

and movements that encourage extension of the thoracic spine are especially useful. Weight-bearing exercises should be high-impact and designed to produce a jarring effect (ground reaction force) greater than twice the client's bodyweight, for example aerobic dance type actions, jogging on a gym treadmill, or weight training.

A number of researchers have illustrated the benefits of weight-bearing exercise in the management of osteoporosis. A 45-minute exercise programme practised over three days per week with postmenopausal women not only slowed loss of bone mineral density but actually showed a 1.4 per cent increase in bone mass during the second and third years of study (Smith *et al*, 1984). A twice-weekly programme of weight-bearing exercise (one hour duration) has been shown to produce a 3.5 per cent increase in bone density of the lumbar spine (Krolner *et al*, 1983).

OSTEOARTHRITIS

Osteoarthritis (or more accurately arthrosis) is a condition associated with both ageing and inactivity, and occurs more commonly where there are biomechanical changes to a joint as a result of past injury. Initially, joint cartilage is affected with changes to its metabolism causing fraying within the periphery of cartilage and later damage (fibrillation) to the deeper cartilage layers. As the condition progresses there may be cartilage blistering and small fragments may break loose and float within the joint (these fragments are called 'loose bodies'). The bone beneath this cartilage layer responds, becoming shiny and smooth (this phenomenon is called eburnation). The joint space reduces as does the movement range. Over time the edge of the bone surface responds by forming small osteophytes, small bone extensions visible on x-ray.

The joint becomes inflamed, and the joint capsule and synovial membrane thicken and increase in vascularity resulting in a higher metabolic rate. Interestingly many of the early changes in arthritis may be reversible, and rehabilitation plays a vital part in this process. Joint loading can change drastically after an injury. For example a change of just 10 per cent in the angle of the knee joint increases the contact force at heel strike from 3.3 times bodyweight up to 7.4 times bodyweight (Sharma *et al*, 2001). It is therefore vital to correct any movement dysfunction in order to re-strengthen a joint following injury.

> **Definition**
>
> Joint space is the distance between the ends of the two bones forming a joint, normally measured using X-rays.

> **Key point**
>
> In arthritis the end of the bone becomes smooth and shiny (eburnation) and small bone spurs (osteophytes) are formed.

Where the spine is affected by arthritis (see fig. 2.5) the facet joints erode and lose their normal smooth surface. The face of the vertebra that is in contact with the disc (the 'vertebral end plate') develops osteophytes – lip-like structures that form on the bone and will be visible on x-rays. These bony spurs can press on nerves and cause direct back pain or referred pain in the buttock or leg. Movement of the spine tends to reduce, especially with regard to rotation, and the spine loses its normal youthful springiness.

The aim of management for spinal arthritis is initially to reduce inflammation, protect the joints and reduce joint loading. This will also reduce pain. A rehab programme can then begin with the aim of re-strengthening the supporting

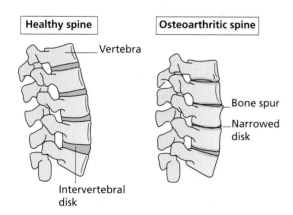

| Healthy spine | Osteoarthritic spine |

Vertebra

Bone spur

Narrowed disk

Intervertebral disk

Figure 2.5 Changes seen in osteoarthritis (OA) of the spine

musculature, initially focusing on core stability, then concentrating on building up strength in the hips and spine. Re-strengthening muscle in this way instigates a process of load sharing where the muscle takes more stress to enable the spinal joints to take less with any given movement. It is perfectly possible to restore full pain-free function using this approach, even though the appearance of the joint on x-ray will be unchanged.

LUMBAGO

'Lumbago' is a catch-all term usually used to describe a dull aching pain in the lumbar spine. Although clearly not a diagnosis it can be useful as it describes the client's condition in a way that is meaningful to them. Someone describing lumbago is most probably indicating that they have a dull ache in their back that does not cause the referred leg pain that would indicate sciatica. Normally lumbago is of muscular origin although conditions affecting the disc and/or facet joints can also cause this type of pain at their outset. The most common cause of lumbago is overuse of the spinal muscles and inflammation of the local tissues, which normally occurs after repeated activity involving bending movements. When tissues become inflamed they display the standard signs of inflammation: redness, heat, swelling and pain (see fig. 2.6). They are sensitive and irritable and easily 'stirred up' by too much movement. Increased local blood flow cause redness and the sensation of heat but, in the case of the spinal tissues, these phenomena may occur too deeply to be seen on the body's surface. Local swelling may be picked up by close observation, but the pressure caused by swelling is often more noticeable, resulting in a sensation of stiffness

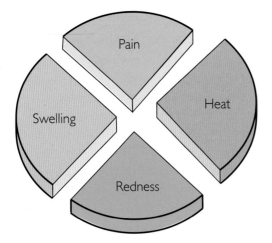

Figure 2.6 Signs of inflammation

and a dull ache in the back. The combination of pain and tissue irritability can cause local spasm to the muscles, and this is a familiar symptom of lumbago.

Initially the aim of treatment is to protect the area and prevent the inflammation from intensifying or spreading to the surrounding tissues. Rest is important provided it is in a supported position (rather than slumped in a chair). Where an individual must continue to work a lumbar support is useful because it enforces rest, reduces motion range and marginally increases intra-abdominal pressure. Most back supports follow a similar design and are wide belts stretching from the inferior aspect of the rib cage to the pelvis. They are elasticated and often secured by velcro fasteners, with plastic or metal stays in the back to prevent or limit lumbar flexion. 'Double pull' belts have a secondary layer of reinforcement, which increases pressure still further. An alternative to the spinal belt is lumbar taping (functional taping). This does not increase intra-abdominal pressure, but instead has a proprioception function, reminding the individual to avoid lumbar flexion. Undertape is placed next to the skin and in most cases elastic taping is placed in strips along the length of the erector spinae muscles (see fig. 2.7).

The initial aim of rehabilitation is to restore range of motion; this is usually done with rotation movements either in sitting or lying. Flexion movements can be used providing they are supported and aim to lengthen the erector spinae muscles. Where the condition has occurred through repeated flexion movements, passive extension is the treatment of choice to target the causal factor. The use of local heat and massage to increase blood flow can be very useful for pain relief, thereby enabling exercise therapy to begin sooner.

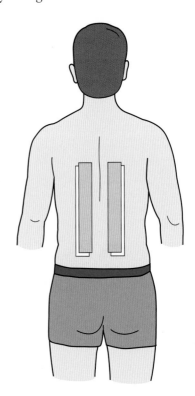

Figure 2.7 Functional taping of the lumbar spine

LUMBAR SURGERY

Rehabilitation forms an essential part of the follow-up to operations on the low back (lumbar surgery). Muscles will need to be re-strengthened, movements regained and functional capacity increased. It is important for therapists and exercise professionals to have a basic overview of the most common types of lumbar surgery in order to make informed choices during rehabilitation and communicate effectively with other health professionals.

The most common types of lumbar surgery (see table 2.1) are those that address the spinal disc. To access the disc the surgeon needs to cut

Table 2.1	Common types of lumbar surgery
Name of operation (surgical procedure)	**What is involved**
Laminectomy	The *lamina* is the part of the bone that joins the spinous process to the transverse process (see fig. 1.1). Part of this bone and the neighbouring *ligamentum flavum* is shaved away to allow access to the damaged spinal discs and affected nerve root. Part of the lamina from the vertebra above the affected area and part of the lamina from the vertebra below is removed. Either some (in a partial laminectomy) or all of the lamina is removed. Where the bony hole surrounding the spinal cord (vertebral foramen) is restricted ('stenosis') this may be enlarged at the same time using a *foraminotomy*.
Microdiscectomy	A portion of the affected disc is removed while a laminectomy is performed. The surgery is performed through a small incision using an operating microscope ('arthroscopic surgery') rather than a larger incision ('open surgery'), so bleeding is lessened and recovery is quicker.
Lumbar fusion	Two or more vertebrae are bound together to create a firm bone pillar, using a bone graft. The bone may be obtained from the patient ('autograft') or a bone bank ('allograft'). 'Posterolateral' fusion puts the graft between the transverse processes while 'interbody' fusion puts the graft in place of the removed spinal disc. No movement is then possible between the operated vertebrae.
Vertebroplasty	A small incision is made and a cement-like substance is inserted into a vertebra under x-ray guidance. The procedure is used in some of the cases of compression fracture that may occur as a result of osteoporosis.
Artificial disc replacement (ADR)	Where a disc has narrowed or collapsed, a disc replacement may be used to maintain disc height. It is sometimes used as an alternative to lumbar fusion.

through the skin and tissue just beneath it (subcutaneous tissue) and often either cut through or split the muscles. In some cases a piece of spinal bone is in the way and some of this may need to be shaved away. The most common piece of bone addressed is the lamina, so the operation is called a laminectomy ('ectomy' meaning to cut away or cut out). This procedure may either involve cutting through the tissues and opening them to see the area to be treated (open surgery) or may be achieved using an operating microscope and very small tools contained within steel tubes (arthroscopic surgery). Less tissue damage occurs in the arthroscopic surgery and so recovery is quicker, but the surgeon's view of the tissues is restricted, so more complex cases involving several tissues may not be suitable for this approach. In some cases the spinal bones may need to be fixed together to form a firm pillar of bone (lumbar fusion). This may be required

Table 2.2	Risks associated with lumbar surgery
Risk	**Explanation**
Reaction to drugs used	All drugs cause changes in the body, but these changes may be unwanted or excessive, in which case they are termed a 'drug reaction'.
Infection	Infection may occur following surgery ('post-operative infection'), necessitating the use of further antibiotics.
Inflammation	Temporary inflammation will occur after spinal surgery but can become prolonged if it affects the membranes surrounding the spinal cord ('arachnoiditis').
Excessive bleeding	Bleeding may occur into the wound site ('haematoma') or into the spinal column ('extradural spinal haematoma').
Nerve damage	Damage to local nerves or the spinal cord itself may occur leading to numbness, muscle weakness or paralysis. This may lead to loss of use in the legs or loss of bladder and bowel control, which may be temporary or permanent.
Failure	Surgery may fail to eliminate symptoms, or fail to achieve what was intended.
Blood clots or stroke	Blood clots may occur in the legs, causing deep vein thrombosis (DVT) or in the lungs causing a pulmonary embolism (PE).
Heart attack	A heart attack may occur as a result of any surgery involving a general anaesthetic, and death can occur. The risk of this is very rare as patients are screened prior to surgery.

Source www.webmd.com, www.nhs.uk.

after disc surgery if further injury occurs, or if the disc surgery is not successful. It can also be used where the spinal bones have been broken (vertebral fracture), as a result of a car accident for example, or in cases of chronic bone thinning (osteoporosis). Nowadays it is possible to replace the spinal disc: either the gel of the disc may be replaced ('nuclear replacement') or the whole disc ('total disc replacement') using a plastic and metal unit.

Any form of surgery has risks, and where larger body areas are treated and/or the operation lasts longer the risk is greater. Risks will be explained before surgery is carried out (see table 2.2), and with modern surgical procedures the risks are relatively few, varying from the minor (such as increased swelling or slight infection) to the more serious (such as blood clots, nerve damage, or a heart attack).

If you are a therapist constructing a rehabilitation programme or a trainer giving a fitness programme to a client who has finished rehab, it is important to seek guidance from your client's surgeon, GP or therapist to identify any restrictions imposed by the surgical procedure. These may include avoiding certain movements or ranges of motion, or reducing spinal loading and weight-bearing.

Key point
Where a client has a history of spinal surgery seek guidance from a medical practitioner or physiotherapist to identify any exercise restrictions.

GENERAL BACK CARE
In chapter 3 we will look at the importance of posture in both standing and sitting, and in chapter 8 at the importance of manual handling techniques as part of functional rehabilitation. Now, however, we will take a brief look at general back care and the actions to take if back pain occurs. When we are performing tasks around the home we often forget the practices that we may use in our general working environment. Repeated actions are an enemy to the spine and it is useful to plan housework and DIY tasks with the spine in mind. Try to avoid repeated stretching when reaching into cupboards or cutting hedges in the garden for example. When reaching to low levels (painting skirting boards for example), kneel rather than stoop into position. Planning heavy lifting tasks is especially important because we probably won't have specialist lifting equipment available in the home as we do within industry. If you know you have a heavy lifting task in the garden it is worth liaising with a neighbour or friend in order to perform two-person lifts rather than struggling by yourself. Repeated actions that involve twisting the spine make it particularly vulnerable and so planning a path to enable us to use our feet to turn our body rather than the spine can be helpful.

When working at your desk at home good ergonomics are as important as they are in the office. Adjusting keyboards, computer monitors, desk layout and chair position are just as important when using a laptop as they are using a desktop computer.

If the spine is injured it is important to rest and support it because trying to work through the pain can cause further problems. Most injuries damage tissue and cause inflammation. Trying to work through an injury can increase both the tissue damage and the body's inflammatory response, causing an exacerbation of symptoms. Resting the spine is better in the lying position, as this places less compression stress on the discs and other spinal tissues. Try to lie on a firm surface with your knees bent to take the stretch off the hip tissues and allow the pelvis and lower spine to orientate correctly. Form a makeshift lumbar support by rolling up a hand towel and placing it into the lumbar lordosis to provide support. When rising from the lying position, turn onto your front, push up onto your hands and knees, draw one knee through, then stand from this position by pressing your hands onto your knee rather than trying to perform a sit-up action on an injured spine (see fig. 2.8). Seek treatment sooner rather than later to prevent a relatively minor injury from turning into a more serious long-term condition.

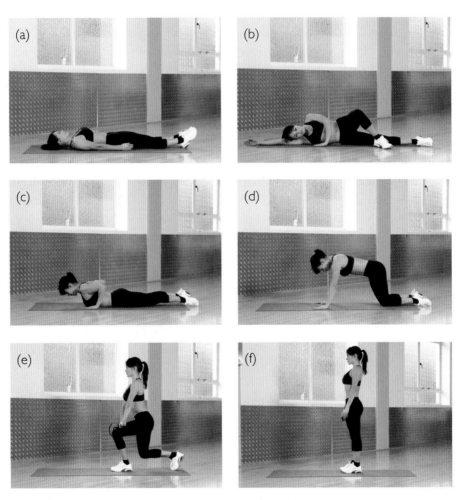

Figure 2.8 Moving from lying down to a standing position

POSTURE AND BACK PAIN

3

Posture is simply the relationship or 'alignment' between the various parts of the body. It is important from two standpoints. Firstly, good posture underlies all exercise techniques. Your posture is really your foundation for movement. In the same way that a building will fall down if its foundations are shaky, your whole body will suffer if your posture is poor. Exercises beginning from the basis of poor posture tend to be awkward and clumsy. Because of this they are less effective and, more importantly, the person undertaking them is more likely to be injured.

The second important point about posture is that an incorrect posture allows physical stress to build up in certain tissues, ultimately leading to pain and injury. For example, a person who is very round-shouldered may simply have started out with tightness in the chest muscles and weakness in the muscles, which brace the shoulders back (see upper crossed syndrome below). If this combination had been corrected at the time, the poor posture would not have built up over the years. The way in which the joints move is altered by poor posture over time. This can result in joints being subjected to uneven stresses. When this continues over the years, the eventual outcome can be the development of wear and tear (osteoarthritis) in later life.

a. Optimal alignment   b. Suboptimal alignment (poor posture)

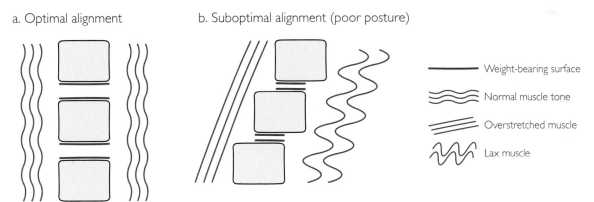

Weight-bearing surface

Normal muscle tone

Overstretched muscle

Lax muscle

Figure 3.1 Poor posture increases pressure on the joint, forcing muscles to work harder

Poor posture gives rise to two key problems. Firstly, joint alignment is not optimal so bodyweight – which would normally be distributed quite evenly across the joints – is taken more by one area than another. This leads to increased stress on portions of the joint (joint loading). Secondly, good posture is a question of balance; very little muscle work is needed to maintain it. With a poor posture the muscles have to work much harder because the body segments are out of alignment. Increased muscle work of this type often leads to aching and can cause painful trigger points within the muscles.

Definition

A trigger point is a painful nodule or taut band lying within a muscle. It is the result of chemical imbalance within the muscle, often due to overwork.

Over time, tissues which are held in a shortened position adapt to become shorter themselves ('adaptive shortening') and those held in a stretched position adapt by becoming longer ('adaptive lengthening'). These changes will happen in all soft tissues, but in different ways. Muscles will respond in the short term by changing their tone (i.e. the way in which they contract) and in the long term by altering their structure. Ligaments, which act to support a joint, will also adapt to changes in joint alignment by becoming longer or shorter over time. Where ligaments are longer, stability of the joint may be compromised, and where they are shorter the range of motion may be reduced.

In chapter 4 we will look in detail at fitness components. In relation to posture, two of the most important fitness components are flexibility (stretching) and strength. Postural changes are often associated with poor muscle tone (weakness) in some muscles together with too much

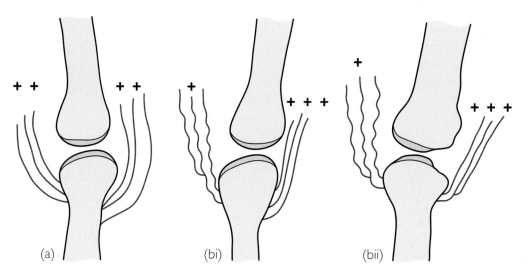

Figure 3.2 Joint mechanics altered by muscle imbalance. (a) normal joint – equal muscle tone gives correct joint alignment; (bi and ii) postural imbalance – unequal muscle tone pulls joint out of ligament

> ## Key point
> With poor posture stress on the joints is increased and the muscles have to work much harder. Over time, tissue adaptation occurs.

> ## Key point
> Your posture will affect the way you exercise, and the exercises you choose will in turn alter your posture.

tone (tightness) in others. This imbalance in tone can cause the muscles around the joint to pull unevenly, causing the joint to move off-centre. One of the aims of exercise is to redress the balance in muscle tone by using stretching exercises to lengthen tight muscles, combined with strengthening exercises at particular joint angles to increase the tone of lax muscles and make them better able to pull the joint closed (inner range). Once this has been achieved, we need to rehearse the correct posture because incorrect posture, when practised over time, becomes a habit ('habitual posture'). In general, strength and stretching exercises are practised as isolated movements, whereas postural rehearsal actions are practised as whole-body actions.

OPTIMAL POSTURE

We cannot talk about a 'normal' posture because very few people are 'normal' in the true sense of the word. Equally, if we talk about an average posture, the average may in fact be very poor. Instead we should talk about an 'optimal' posture, where the various body segments are aligned correctly, and minimum stress is placed on the body tissues. This type of posture requires little muscle activity to maintain, because it is essentially balanced, and so is more energy efficient.

The various segments of the body work together like the links in a chain. Movement in one causes movement in the next, which is then passed on to the next and so on. This means that a postural change in one part of the body can alter the alignment of another body part quite far away. Alterations in the feet are a good illustration of this point. Flat feet, where the inner arch of the foot drops downwards, will in turn twist the shinbone and then the thighbone. Eventually these changes can be felt in the lower back, chest and neck. Because of this intimate link between body segments, it is important to correct any postural fault, however minor it may at first seem.

> ## Key point
> In an optimal posture the body segments are correctly aligned, so very little effort is needed to maintain the position.

ASSESSING POSTURE IN THE CLINIC

Posture may be labelled 'static' (still) or 'dynamic' (moving). Static posture looks at one body segment relative to another along a vertical posture line (gravity line). This type of assessment uses a plumb line and/or posture chart and can suggest areas where further testing is required. For example, shortened tissue may develop trigger points requiring more attention from a soft-tissue therapist, while lengthened tissue may respond to exercise designed to shorten muscle fibres (these are called 'inner-range actions').

Dynamic posture can give information about the alignment of the segments of the body, but also deals with muscle actions and motor skill. In the clinic we are mainly interested in walking, bending and sitting, as these are functional actions used in day-to-day life. In sport, actions such as running, jumping and throwing are examples of clinically important dynamic postures. A keen clinical eye may be used to view dynamic posture, but the speed of an action means that video and computer equipment are very useful, and the cost of these systems is reducing all the time. A simple video camera on a tripod or a mobile phone can often yield important information for both the therapist and client, and there are even smart-phone apps to help with assessment. The advent of pinch-to-zoom and freeze-frame on smart-phone and tablet screens means the therapist can focus on a specific body area to facilitate client education. As the proverb says, 'a picture paints a thousand words', this is especially true in the case of posture re-education.

> ### Key point
> Static posture assesses body alignment at rest, dynamic posture assesses alignment during movement.

FROM THE SIDE
Static posture assessment begins with the subject standing behind a plumb line or posture screen. A simple plumb line can be constructed using a length of string with a small weight tied on the end, and a posture screen can be made using a 1.5 x 2 m piece of firm plastic sheeting with grid lines drawn with a magic marker pen.

From the side the posture line should pass just in front of the ankle bone ('lateral malleolus'), just in front of the centre of the knee joint, through the greater trochanter of the hip, then the bodies of the lumbar vertebrae and the centre of the shoulder joint and ear. This line is not set purely at random. The line was described in the 1950s by researchers who weighed body segments to find the centre of gravity of each. By joining the centres of each body part into a model of the full body, the posture line was established.

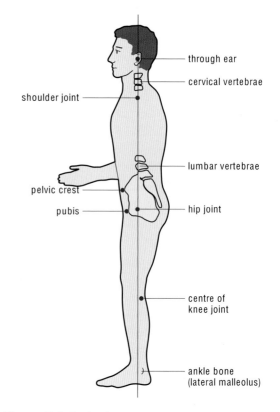

Figure 3.3 Optimal posture

Because the posture line passes through the centre of the knee joint, the knee is pressed straight and locks ('extensor torque'), meaning that you do not require any muscle activity in your quadriceps to remain standing upright. If the knee moves forward, the line passes behind the centre of the knee causing the knee to bend and unlock (flexor torque); this action must be resisted by activity in the quads. This muscle activity has two effects: firstly, it is tiring over time, and secondly, the patella is pressed onto the patellar surface of the femur below. This can worsen the condition of someone suffering from patellofemoral pain.

Also, to compare the knee alignment for both sides, go round to the other side of your client. The ankle, knee and hip should be in line. It is common to see one or both knees behind or in front of the line between the ankle and hip. Where the knee lies in front of the leg line, it has not locked out. This may often occur following injury, especially where the knee is swollen. As the knee extends for the last few degrees the knee bones twist and the tightness of the knee ligaments locks the knee (this is called the 'screw home effect'). This stabilises the knee so that no muscle work is required to stand with the leg locked in this way. However, if the knee fails to lock completely the screw home effect will not occur and the knee will have to be stabilised by continuous muscle work – a much more demanding situation. Where the knee lies behind the leg line ('genu recurvatum') the knee has hyperextended overstretching its posterior structures. Bear in mind that any change in leg alignment can alter walking or running gait and have an indirect effect on either the pelvis or lumbar spine. For this reason, lower limb alignment is important when planning back rehabilitation.

The position of the greater trochanter, pelvis and lumbar spine is important for low back pain. We saw in chapter 1 that the pelvis balances like a seesaw with the hip joints as pivots. The guide wires that control pelvic position are the muscles and soft tissues attaching to the bones. These include the abdominals and hip flexors at the front and the spinal extensors and gluteal (buttock) muscles at the back. Postural changes will alter the tilt of the pelvis and change the resting length of these muscles. Over time some muscles shorten and tighten, while others lengthen and become lax. The result is muscle imbalance. When the pelvis tips forwards (anterior pelvic tilt) the lumbar curve (lordosis) will increase, hollowing the back. When it tips backwards (posterior pelvic tilt) the back is flattened. In each case there is an alteration in the stress imposed on the spinal tissues, discs and facet joints. In an optimal posture the pelvis remains level, with the lines through the anterior superior iliac spine (ASIS) at the front of the pelvis and posterior superior iliac spine (PSIS) at the back being roughly horizontal. The range of normal values of anterior is between zero and five degrees. In addition, the ASIS should be in the same vertical alignment as the pubis. Where alignment of these vertical and horizontal lines of the pelvis is optimal, the lumbar curve (lordosis) is shallow and even.

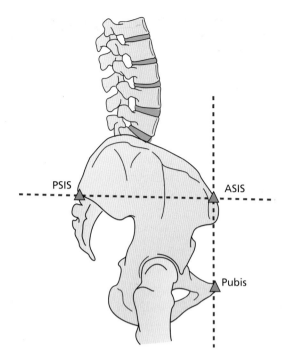

Figure 3.4 Horizontal and vertical alignment of the pelvis in optimal posture

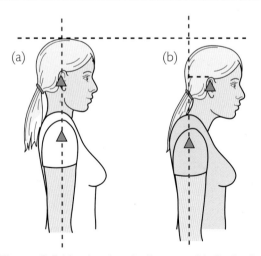

Figure 3.5 Head and neck alignment. (a) Optimal – head and neck alignment over shoulder. (b) Sub optimal – head centre forwards of shoulder creating extra leverage force

The shoulder should lie on the posture line in an optimal posture, but commonly it is pulled forward due to slouching in sitting and driving postures throughout our daily lives. This body position can lead to tightness in the anterior shoulder and chest muscles. A forward-lying shoulder posture can also be the result of increased curvature of the thoracic spine (thoracic kyphosis), forward tilting of the scapula, or anterior shifting of the head of the humerus (ball) within the glenoid cavity at the shoulder joint (socket). Often several factors coexist, so close examination of your client is vital to ensure treatment is targeted at the right structures.

The ear should rest on the posture line, with the neck forming a shallow inward curve (cervical lordosis). One of the most common postural abnormalities is that of the forward head posture, where the head is thrust forwards, increasing cervical lordosis. Because the ear has now moved forwards of the posture line a leverage force has been introduced, effectively increasing the weight of the head. This increased head weight requires additional muscle work to hold the neck in position, and results in tightening of the sub occipital muscles and laxity of the neck flexors.

FROM BEHIND

From behind, the posture line should bisect the body into two symmetrical halves (see table 3.1). From the ground the spread of the heel tissue

Table 3.1	Assessing standing posture from behind		
Part of the body	**Changes**	**Part of the body**	**Changes**
Ear level/hair line		Skin creases	
Shoulder level – cervical spine		Levels of pelvic rim, ASIS, belt line	
Inferior angle of scapula		Buttock creases	
Overall spinal alignment		Knee creases/muscle bulk	
Keyhole		Mid-line/Achilles angle	
Adam's position		Foot position	

43

and height of the foot arches should be equal. The Achilles' tendon should be vertical and have an equal hollow on each side. The depth of the foot arches should also be the same for both sides of the body. An easy way to quickly assess arch height is to locate the navicular bone at the highest point of the inside (medial) arch. You should be able to place one thumb between the navicular bone and the floor. If you are unable to get your thumb into the gap the arch is too low and the foot is flattened ('Pes Planus') and if you can get both thumbs in the gap, the arch is too high and the foot is hollowed ('Pes Cavus').

The arch height and Achilles' alignment often change in conjunction with one another, so closer assessment of the whole area may be required. Look at your client walking and see the imprint that their foot makes on the floor. Changes in foot position directly affect lower limb alignment, which in turn alters the level of stress imposed on the lumbar spine. The reverse can also occur, and pain and movement dysfunction in the lumbar spine can cause alteration in gait patterns and changes in foot position.

Calf bulk should be the same on each side with the knee creases level and kneecaps facing in the same direction. Look for symmetry of muscle bulk. It is common for one calf to be larger than the other, especially following an injury, and the angulation of the patellae can suggest changes in patella position relative to the underlying femur, or rotation of the leg from the hip or foot. Remember also that where nerve impingement occurs within the lumbar spine, nervous impulses travelling through the nerves in the legs will be impaired. Impairment of the motor nerve can cause muscle wasting over time, and requires referral to a physiotherapist.

Asymmetry of the lumbar musculature is common. Muscle wasting following long-term pain may occur, while short-term pain may result from muscle spasm. Ask your client to bend forward while you squat down to look across their back muscles (the 'skyline view', also known as 'Adam's position') at waist level. The rounded contour of the spine can sometimes help you detect more subtle contour changes. Changes in rib position can also be seen in this position higher up the body in the thoracic region.

Where asymmetry is noted in the spinal extensor muscle, side bending is likely to be restricted away on the thinner side (e.g. if the muscles are tight on the left side, bending will be reduced on the right side). Tightness and shortness in the soft tissues on one side of the body may also pull the spine away from the vertical position, altering the position of the shoulders relative to the pelvis. If this change is very subtle it may be difficult to detect, but noting

(a) (b)

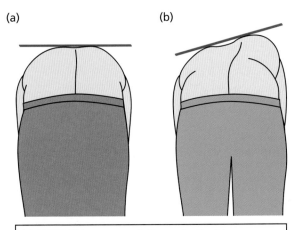

(a) NORMAL – curve of ribs on both sides of the body equal. Spine straight.
(b) ABNORMAL – curve of rib on right side of body higher, spine curved to side (scoliosis).

Figure 3.6 Changes in rib position

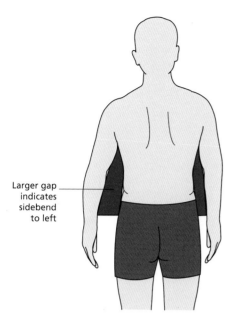

Larger gap indicates sidebend to left

Figure 3.7 The keyhole between the arm and body

Definition

The acromion process is the bony protrusion on the shoulder blade.

Key point

The trapezius muscles connect the base of the skull, the shoulder blades and the lower thoracic vertebrae.

Definition

The sternocleidomastoid muscle is a paired muscle at the surface of the front of the neck.

the gap between the arm and side of the body (called the 'keyhole') can make things easier. If the trunk is pulled to the left, the right arm will fall closer to the body (narrower keyhole) while the left falls further away (wider keyhole). Tightness which extends into the quadratus lumborum muscles at the side of the spine will also anchor the lower ribs down, reducing the gap between the pelvic rim and lower ribs. Again, compare one side to the other: the thicker, shorter muscle is normally on the side of reduced space.

Moving up to the thoracic region each scapula should lie approximately one hand-width from the spine. A closer position can indicate shortening in the rhomboid muscles between the scapulae, while a position further away normally indicates tightness in the pectoral muscles of the chest and laxity of the shoulder retractor muscles. The contour of the shoulder shows the

relative condition of the upper trapezius, with a rigid cord-like contour indicating an overly tight, thickened muscle. A line drawn between the acromion processes of each side should be horizontal. Tightness of the trapezius and sternocleidomastoid muscles can cause the shoulder to raise, while laxity of these muscles and poor scapular stability can cause the scapula (shoulder blade) and clavicle to drop, a common feature in thoracic outlet syndrome (TOS), which causes neurological pain to be referred from the shoulder into the arm.

FROM THE FRONT

Posture assessment from the front looks mainly at symmetry of muscle development and ribcage alignment. Begin by looking at ankle and foot alignment to confirm your findings from postural evaluation from the side and back. Next, look at the thigh muscles (quadriceps) as asymmetry and wasting is common in those with a history of knee injury. Note also the gap between the knees to determine if your client has knock knees (genu valgum) or bowlegs (genu varum). Normally the bones of the inner knee (medial condyle) and the bones of the inner ankle (medial malleolus) of each side should be close together.

The pelvis and hips should be in horizontal alignment when viewed from the front, with the greater trochanters in line and the ASIS of each side also in line. Commonly, one hip may drop, showing the greater trochanter lowering on that side, with the pelvis tipping away from the horizontal. Two main causes are common here: leg length discrepancy and change in hip muscle balance. Leg length changes can occur where the femur or tibia of one side are of unequal length. This may be developmental or as a result of trauma. As babies many of our bones are relatively soft. As we grow the bones harden (ossify), until

during adolescence we are left with bones which have just a small cartilage growth at the ends (this is called the 'epiphyseal plate'). The growth plate is the only region of the bone that now grows, and any damage to a growth plate, through injury or a medical condition, will stop the bone growing any further.

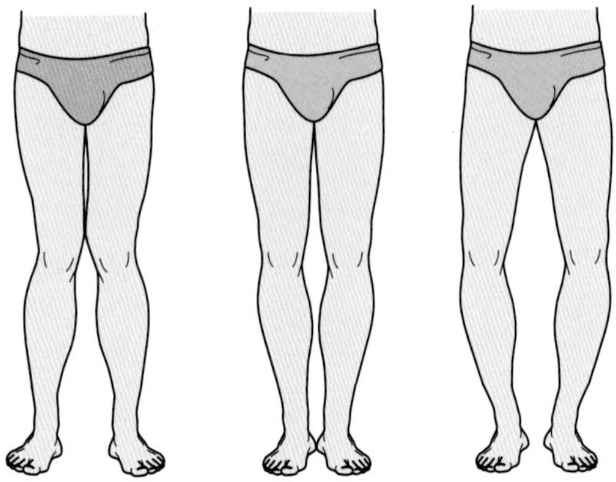

Severe trauma, such as a broken leg as a result of a road traffic accident, can lead to bones healing slightly shorter than they were, so if your client has had this type of injury, one leg may well be shorter than the other and they will need a built-up shoe. Clinical measures of leg length are available and the client should be referred to an orthopaedic specialist for this, as significant changes in leg length will cause a low-level but continuous stress on the spine.

Changes in leg alignment may also occur following hip pain. The side gluteal muscles (gluteus medius) hold the pelvis up when you stand on one leg. If this muscle is weak (common in the swayback posture described below) the pelvis will drop downwards when your client stands on one leg (a *positive* Trendelenburg sign). Over time this type of asymmetry of muscle strength may lead to an alteration of posture even when standing on both legs. Your client may favour one leg and shift their pelvis over that side with little weight taken on the other side. In addition, to compensate for the horizontal tip in the pelvis the clients

Genu valgum	Normal alignment	Genu varum
Knees closer together than ankles	Ankles and knees equal distance apart	Ankles closer together than knees

Figure 3.8 Leg alignment in postural assessment

Definition

A positive Trendelenburg sign occurs when the subject's pelvis drops when they stand on one leg, indicating that they have weak or paralysed hip muscles.

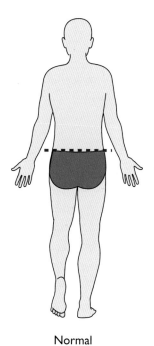

Normal

Pelvis level with both legs
on the ground. Remains level
when one leg bends

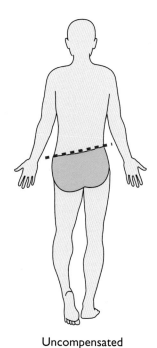

**Uncompensated
Trendelenburg signs**

Pelvis tipped with both legs
on the ground. Trunk remains
vertical when one leg bends

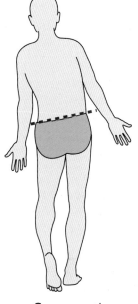

**Compensated
Trendelenburg signs**

Pelvis tipped with both legs
on the ground. Trunk side
bends when one leg bends

Figure 3.9 Pelvic alignment in standing position

trunk may bend to the side, shortening the trunk tissues on one side and lengthening them on the other, giving the appearance of a side bent spine or scoliosis.

Definition

A scoliosis is a side bending of the spine. Structural scoliosis occurs due to changes in spinal bone shape, functional scoliosis due to changes in the length of muscle or other soft tissue.

The ribcage should be symmetrical, but a number of changes may be seen here as well. The lower ribs should be on the same horizontal line. Where they are not, the spine may be tipped to the side or the side flexor muscles may be tighter on one side, requiring stretching (see below). Palpation will be necessary, because some individuals have one fewer rib on one side than the other.

The sternum (breastbone) should be vertical or angled upwards slightly. Thoracic flexion (increased kyphosis) will angle the sternum down, and some individuals have a developmentally altered sternal alignment. A funnel chest (pectus excavatum) is a condition where there is too much connective tissue attaching the ribs to the sternum, causing the sternum to be pressed inwards.

The clavicles should be symmetrical, and frequently changes in the scapula identified during postural assessment from behind are confirmed by looking from the front as well. Finally the head should be held straight, with tightness in the upper trapezius or sternocleidomastoid muscles typically presenting as a raised shoulder and/or sideways-tipped head. Tightness in these muscles will often restrict rotation and side flexion movements of the head. Where restriction to active movement is found (ask your client to turn their head or take their ear towards their shoulder as far as they can) relax the tight muscle by raising the shoulder blade (shrugging). If movement range to the head and neck is increased in this way, muscle tightness is confirmed as a limiting factor.

POSTURAL SWAY

Although we assess static posture, when standing upright, the human body is not in fact stationary. Due to the small base of support (surface area of the feet) and relatively high centre of gravity located within the sacrum, the body resembles a tall block standing on end. As such it is inherently unstable, and in order to remain upright, there is a continuous motion called postural sway. The body moves forwards and backwards through activity of the calf and shin muscles, and side to side through shifting of the pelvis. This alternating muscle activity provides a relief mechanism to reduce fatigue in the legs and aid blood flow through the accessory muscle pump. Body sway is greater in taller and heavier individuals, and

increases following injury and during old age. In addition, body sway has been shown to increase in clients with chronic low back pain. Rehabilitation programmes can be targeted to reduce body sway following injury, or to reduce the risk of a fall in the elderly.

USING POSTURE CHARTS

Posture charts help you to record your client's static posture from the side ('sagittal plane') and behind ('frontal plane'). For observations from in front, additional clinical notes can be made. For each body segment the line figure reminds you of what to look for, and you can score your clients posture 3 (good: optimal), 2 (intermediate: slightly suboptimal) or 1 (poor: gross changes). Although subjective, the numbering system gives your client a 'posture value' with a maximum value of 48 and a minimum of 16, and this can be converted to a percentage by placing their value over 48 as a fraction and multiplying by 100. For example a client who scores a total of 24 gets a posture value of 50 per cent (24/48 x 100), and someone scoring 35 gets a value of 73 per cent (35/48 x 100). The posture value can then be used to track progress of therapy to optimise a client's posture.

GENERAL PRINCIPLES OF POSTURAL EXERCISE

To modify posture using exercise therapy, we must stretch tight muscle to allow correct movement to take place. If we simply try to exercise against a tight muscle it becomes self-defeating: the exercise tries to move the body in one direction and the body simply pulls itself back! Once we have stretched and free movement is possible, we now can shorten a lax muscle. This has the effect of holding the body part in the correct position. Stretching and strengthening (muscle shortening) in this way begins to correct the muscle imbalance that is usually the key feature of postural changes. However, changing the body tissues in this way will allow us to move correctly, but we still may not choose to do so. This is because the suboptimal posture has been present for some time and has become familiar (like a bad habit) hence the term habitual posture. To modify this, we must continually practise correct exercise postures to rehearse optimal posture and break bad habits.

POSTURE OPTIMISATION
SUBOPTIMAL POSTURE IN THE LUMBO-PELVIC REGION

When assessing posture from the side using a plumb line, four posture types are commonly seen. *Flatback*, *swayback*, and *lordotic* reflect the alignment of the pelvis relative to the lumbar spine. *Kyphotic* posture shows the alignment of the thoracic spine. The postural changes seen around the pelvic girdle and shoulder girdle were termed 'crossed syndromes' by the famous Czech rehabilitation specialist Vladimir Janda. The crossed syndrome affecting the lower spine, is called the lower (pelvic) crossed syndrome (LCS) and that affecting the upper spine, the upper (scapular) crossed syndrome (UCS). Each crossed syndrome is so-called because of the combination of laxity and tightness in opposing muscles on the front and back of the body. The lower crossed syndrome results from lengthening of the abdominal and gluteal muscles, in combination with tightness in the lower back and hip flexor muscles. The upper crossed syndrome results from a combination of tightening in the chest musculature and muscles

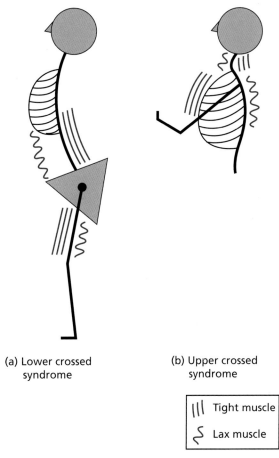

(a) Lower crossed syndrome

(b) Upper crossed syndrome

| ||| | Tight muscle |
| ⌇ | Lax muscle |

Figure 3.10 Crossed syndrome

attaching to the skull base (upper trapezius and suboccipitals) with laxity of the shoulder retractors and cervical flexors.

Although each posture type has distinct features, clinically there is often overlap between the types and subgroups within each category. The names of these combinations indicate their root types, for example kypho-lordotic, asymmetrical swayback, high lordotic and low lordotic. Where combinations are found, therapy is modified depending on clinical findings and the client's reaction to treatment.

In an optimal posture the greater trochanter of the femur lies on the posture line when viewed from the side. The pelvis remains level, with a line through the anterior superior iliac spine (ASIS) and posterior superior iliac spine (PSIS) being roughly horizontal (5° anterior tilt). In this optimal position the lumbar curve (lordosis) is shallow and even. If you take your client to a wall, and position them with their shoulders (scapulae) and back (sacrum) bones pressed against the wall, you should be able to get the flat of your hand between the wall and their flesh. If you can't get your hand into the gap, their lordosis is shallower than normal (flatback). On the other hand if you can get your whole fist in the gap their lordosis is deeper than normal (lordotic). The depth of the lordosis will reflect the alignment of the individual spinal bones (vertebrae). We saw in chapter 1 that the vertebrae contact each other via the spongy spinal disc at the front and two facet joints at the back. Increasing the lordosis tips one vertebra backwards relative to its neighbour (extension) while reducing the lordosis tips one vertebra forwards (flexion). In each case the stress imposed on the discs and facet joints will change as the depth of the lordosis alters.

FLATBACK POSTURE

In a flatback posture the pelvis remains level or is slightly posteriorly tilted, but the most important feature is the reduction or loss of the lumbar lordosis. Looking at a client from the side, there is no longer an inward curve in the lumbar spine, and in extreme cases the lumbar spine may be flexed further, with the client appearing bent forwards and frequently placing their hands on their thighs to support themselves when rising to standing from sitting.

Effectively each lumbar vertebra becomes slightly flexed relative to its neighbour, opening the facet joints at the back slightly and compressing the spinal disc at the front. On closer examination the loss of lordosis may be more noticeable in the upper or lower lumbar spine. The distinction into upper or lower regions occurs due to the postural stress, which has been imposed on the spine. When lumbar flexion is led by posterior pelvic tilt (sitting or drawing the knees to the chest) the lumbar spine flexes from below upwards, so L5 (5th moves before L4 and L3. Where lumbar flexion is led by forward bending (stooping and lifting actions) lumbar flexion occurs from above (L1 moving before L2 and L3). The former stress (sitting) tends to flatten the lower lumbar curve, the latter stress (stooping) flattens the upper lumbar curve.

A client with a flatback posture will often have a history of low back pain. Pain is generally made worse when the flatback posture is exacerbated by bending activities such as housework, DIY, or gardening.

In the flatback posture the lumbar spine is effectively flexed, so extension movements should be used to correct it. However, where pain is high (6–8 on a VAS – Visual analogue scale) we may choose to use rotation actions to begin with in order to free up the back and reduce spasming. This process is begun with manual therapy. Exercise therapy focuses on two exercises initially: passive spinal extension, also called extension in lying (EIL) and pelvic tilting described in chapter 6.

LORDOTIC POSTURE

In a lordotic posture the lumbar lordosis (inward curve) is increased and the pelvis anteriorly tilted so that the ASIS is substantially lower than the PSIS. Again this may occur in upper or lower portions, with obesity and lax abdominal muscles tending to give a lower lordotic posture, while an upper lordotic posture is often associated with a swayback posture (see below).

The classical imbalance of the lordotic posture is lengthening of the abdominal muscles with shortening of the hip flexor muscles – the lower crossed syndrome mentioned above. The erector spinae muscles tighten and shorten and the gluteal muscles often waste. During rehabilitation, soft tissue therapy is aimed at reducing pain within the erector spinae and encouraging contraction of the gluteals using muscle facilitation techniques (see chapter 6) .

Exercise therapy for lordotic posture

We can begin exercise therapy for a lordotic posture by encouraging flexion. The aim here is twofold. The ultimate goal is to reduce the depth of the lordosis. This will involve both passive and resisted actions to reduce stiffness and address muscle weakness and lengthening. At the initial stage, however, flexion aims to combat the extension stress, which may be causing pain.

Supported lumbar flexion is used at this stage, with the patient either lying and drawing the knees to the chest (lower lumbar spine) or standing and flexing the spine while taking the bodyweight through the arms, both described in chapter 6.

The lordotic posture is a combination of stiffness in the spinal joints and tissues and muscle imbalance. The two exercises above target lumbar stiffness and reduced motion range. Now we need to look at muscle imbalance. Often when a person has had an injury or a painful condition for a long time we tend to think of muscle weakness and joint stiffness as important factors. Clearly this is the case, but from the point of view of muscle condition, some muscles tend to lose tone and become lax and lengthened, while others increase their tone and become tight and shorter. We need to address this imbalance rather than simply working all muscles equally. The lordotic posture is called lower crossed syndrome because it often combines laxity in the abdominal muscles (especially the lower abdominals) and gluteals, with tightness or shortness in the hip flexors and spinal extensors.

To shorten lengthened muscles we need to work them at their inner range against resistance. Inner range (i.e. when a joint is closed) shortens the muscle by drawing its actin and myosin filaments together. By rehearsing this action repeatedly the body learns to reset the muscle (neural control) and is able to hold the muscle in inner range more easily. Two exercises are important, pelvic tilting against a wall and the modified trunk curl (see chapter 6).

The lordotic posture is also associated with two clinical conditions: obesity and childbirth. Correction of the lordotic posture in an obese client has to be carried out in parallel with dietary advice for weight loss. The increased mass of the abdominal wall caused by fat deposition in obesity causes the abdomen to protrude forwards and downwards.

This movement draws the abdominal contents downwards (visceral ptosis), and in some cases the rectus abdominis muscle can split centrally allowing the contents to protrude through the muscle at times of abdominal strain, when intra-abdominal pressure is increased. This condition can be clinically important as weakness in this area increases risk of a hernia.

During pregnancy, the developing child creates a similar mass on the front and lower abdomen. The weight is again pulled forwards and downwards, but as the child's weight increases during the third trimester of pregnancy, the abdominal muscles have a shorter time to adapt than they do with the obese client. For this reason the abdominal muscles do not stretch to as great an extent in pregnancy as they do in obesity. Splitting of the rectus abdominis (diastasis) may still occur but will usually be reversed spontaneously following childbirth. A significant difference in the pelvic condition during pregnancy when compared to obesity is the softening of the pelvic joints caused by the release of female hormones. Softening of the pubis and sacroiliac joints occurs to facilitate childbirth and again should resolve spontaneously following birth of the baby. In cases where this does not occur referral to a physiotherapist is vital.

SWAYBACK POSTURE

In the lordotic posture the greater trochanter stays on the posture line but the pelvis is tilted. With the swayback posture the pelvis remains more or less level, but the whole pelvis is thrust forward so that the greater trochanter lies anterior to the posture line. In an optimal posture the sternum is the most anterior bony point of the body, but with a swayback posture the ASIS is the most anterior. The swayback is often called the 'slouched' posture as it occurs with prolonged standing when relaxed. Essentially the client is balancing on the elasticity of their anterior hip tissues, and the posture often favours one leg (asymmetrical swayback). Now, if the left leg is locked out straight and the right is bent at the knee, the client presses their pelvis forward and to the left placing their bodyweight over the straight leg. The body is now supported by the hip abductor muscles of the straight (left) leg and the elasticity of the anterior hip structures of the same leg. The bent (right) leg plays little part in taking bodyweight, acting more for balance.

It is clear that this posture will cause problems because one leg takes most of the person's bodyweight over a long period. Hip and knee pain are the most frequently observed symptoms, with the powerful hip abductor muscles (gluteus medius) becoming fatigued and the client relying on the tensor fascia lata (TFL) muscle and iliotibial band (ITB) instead. The ITB presses against the greater trochanter at the hip and the lateral epicondyle at the knee sometimes giving rise to ITB friction syndrome.

The position of the spine is one of extension and side flexion (or more accurately, side shifting), leading to shortening of tissue on one side and lengthening on the other. When viewed from behind, the lower ribs and pelvis appear closer together on the side with the shortened side flexor muscles. Soft tissue therapy may be used to release the tight tissue and should be followed by stretching to regain tissue length. As the swayback is often an asymmetrical posture, exercise therapy begins with asymmetrical movements as well. Supported side bend actions over a bench and side shift actions against a wall are useful to lengthen the shortened tissues on one side of the body (see chapter 6).

KYPHOTIC POSTURE

Within the thoracic region postural changes occur in the scapulae and thoracic curve, as the two are intimately connected. Optimally, the scapulae lie three finger widths from the spine with their straight medial border vertical. The inferior angle of the scapula typically lies level with T7 (the seventh thoracic vertebra), the root of the scapular spine with T4 and the superior angle with T1. Modern life sees us working at desks, using tools and driving, all activities that require us to flex and adduct the arms. As a result the scapula often move apart and away from the midline (this is called 'scapular abduction'). At the same time they may rotate downwards, causing the glenoid cavity to point towards the floor. This posture has important implications for coordinated movement of the scapula and humerus, and is a risk factor for shoulder impingement conditions (see Norris (2011) *The Complete Guide to Sports Injuries*, pp. 149–159). The forward motion of the scapula draws the whole weight of the arm forwards and away from the posture line, increasing the arm's leverage effect. The result is that the thoracic spine follows this motion and flexes, increasing the curvature of the thoracic kyphosis causing the classic kyphotic posture.

> **Definition**
> The glenoid cavity is the shallow cavity that forms a joint with the humerus.

The adducted, downward-rotated position of the scapulae in the kyphotic posture places stress on the rhomboid muscles and levator scapulae. These muscles often develop trigger points which respond well to soft tissue therapy, paralleled with exercise to retract and stabilise the scapulae and press the thoracic spine into extension.

> **Definition**
> The rhomboid muscles are the rhombus-shaped muscles attached to the scapula, they are primarily responsible for retracting the shoulder blade. The levator scapulae are muscles found at the side and rear of the neck. Their principal function is lifting the shoulder blade.

Where pain occurs in the overstretched tissues taping can be used to unload the affected tissues. (see Norris, *Complete Guide to Sports Injuries*, 2011, for taping details).

Exercise therapy is used to correct the flexed thoracic position. The sternal lift exercise is a useful action where the client draws the scapulae down and together, while lifting the sternum and straightening the thoracic spine. Where the thoracic spine is very stiff, passive stretching over a roll or gym ball may be used to extend the thoracic spine and open up the ribcage (chapter 6).

SITTING POSTURE

Maintaining a neutral lumbar position is also important in sitting. We spend much of our working day sitting at computers and driving, and a suboptimal sitting position can place considerable stress on the spine. The neutral position of the spine is the one that places the least stress on the lumbar tissues, and when we move out of this position stress is imposed onto the anteriorly or posteriorly placed structures. The position of the lumbar spine and depth of the lumbar lordosis is closely interrelated to the angle of the pelvic tilt. As we move from standing to sitting, the hips flex and force the pelvis to posteriorly rotate. The point at which this occurs is dependent on body proportions and tissue flexibility, but in general we can expect posterior pelvic rotation to have occurred by the time the knee has reached hip level (i.e. when the femur is 90° to the bodyline). Tilting can occur in some subjects within the first third of hip flexion motion (0–60°) and in others not until the start of the final third (120°). Clearly, sitting on a low chair imposes a greater stress on the spine as the hip flexion angle is increased and the lumbar lordosis reduced.

Maintenance of normal lumbar lordosis is dependent on the knee being positioned below the hip, and a lumbar support being built into the chair where the spine rests on the chair back. Many individuals will move forward to the front edge of the chair so that the ischial tuberosities rest on the chair base but the pubic bones are anterior to the chair seat. This position encourages anterior pelvic tilt and the maintenance of a normal lordosis.

Often high-quality office chairs and car seats have a built-in adjustable lumbar support. These can be raised or lowered to accommodate different body heights and spinal links and also alter

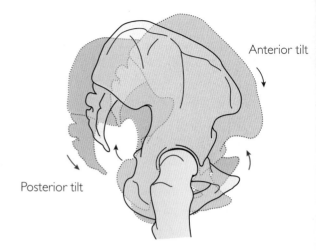

Figure 3.11 Pelvic tilt in sitting

in depth to suit different individual needs. Where lumbar support is not built into the chair it can be added in the form of a lumbar roll. If these are not available a temporary solution is to roll a hand towel and place it in the lumbar lordosis resting just above the trouser belt line.

The general position of the lower spine has a knock-on effect on head and neck position. A flexed spinal position in sitting will lead to a head-forward posture, placing additional stress on the neck tissues. This type of posture can lead to tension across the shoulders (trapezius muscle) and into the neck (trapezius, sternocleidomastoid and cervical extensors).

PRINCIPLES OF BACK REHABILITATION 4

Back rehabilitation has a number of aims. Firstly to restrengthen weakened muscles, secondly to regain lost mobility and thirdly to restore function where movement dysfunction has occurred. The term 'movement dysfunction' takes in both physical and psychological aspects including motor programmes and fear of movement. Restoring range of motion involves both the spine itself and the limb muscles attaching to the pelvic girdle and shoulder girdle. To understand spinal restrengthening we need to have an appreciation of the way in which the spine is supported, that is to say its stabilisation mechanisms.

STABILISATION MECHANISMS OF THE LUMBAR SPINE

If we can maintain the neutral position of the spine when we move or lift, for example, we can greatly reduce the stress on the spinal tissues. This is an essential part of the concept of core stability (back stability).

The concept of holding one part firm so that another part can move effectively is not new, of course, and is seen in all sorts of common daily activities. When we drive a car, for example, we put our foot on the accelerator and expect the car to

Definition

Core stability means holding the centre of the body still to act as a firm base for the arms and legs to move on.

go forward. For this to happen, the tyre must grip on the road surface and the road must stay firm or 'stable'. If the tyre is in contact with ice, the wheel simply spins and the car cannot move forward. A similar mechanism can be said to occur with the spine. In the case of the lumbar spine, a lack of stability will cause energy to be wasted on moving the spine. This can be conserved in overhead press actions in the gym when the lumbar spine is unstable. Looking at the lumbar spine, the lumbar curvature (lordosis) is seen to increase dramatically as someone presses the weight bar overhead. Similarly, when an individual moves their arm, the humerus should move on the stable scapula. If the scapular stabilisers are not working correctly, some of the energy which should go into lifting the arm will be lost if the scapula moves around the rib cage instead. In both cases failure of the stabilising muscles has made the movement less efficient and caused a part of the body to move unnecessarily.

INTERACTING COMPONENTS OF STABILITY

The core of the body is the part between the pelvis and the ribcage. The axial skeleton consists of the spine and ribcage, the appendicular skeleton the limbs, pelvis and scapulae. The essential principle of spinal stability is that muscles should work to hold the axial skeleton firmly and allow the appendicular skeleton to move on a stable base. Core stability results from the interplay between three body components. The first is the shape of the bones and joints. This is called the 'passive' component because it is moved by forces outside the body, such as heavy weight, but is not able to move by itself. If the passive system breaks down, the body's core will lose stability. A broken bone or dislocated joint, for example, will leave the body virtually unable to move because the body part is insecure. No matter how much we pull or push on it, pain and instability will stop us moving effectively. The body recognises what will damage us and forces us to rest.

The next component that contributes to core stability is the 'active' system. This is made up of the muscles, which pull on the bones and joints, either to hold them firm or to move them. In order to do this effectively, the muscles must be sufficiently strong. Using the example of the broken bone above, if we place the limb in a plaster cast the bone will heal: the 'passive' system (bone) therefore becomes more stable. However, when we remove the plaster cast all the muscles will have wasted and we are too weak to move the limb very far or hold it firm. This is why after a fracture the leg often 'gives way' when we twist or turn suddenly. The passive stability (bone) is fine, but the active stability (muscle) is weak.

When the muscles become strong again, we cannot use them all the time because they will get tired, and we do not want contantly tense muscles. The ideal situation is to be able to turn the muscles on and off so that we can use them to stabilise the body when we need them to and allow them to rest when we don't. Economy of movement is the key here, and this is the job of the third stability component, 'control'. This system works by the brain and spinal cord monitoring tiny sensors in the joints and muscles of the body called proprioceptors. These sensors give us information about body position, movement and the stress imposed on the body through everyday activities. When a joint or body part is put under strain, the proprioceptors will detect this and send a message to the muscles to tighten and hold that part of the body firm to resist the forces stressing it.

Key point

Core stability relies on passive (bone and ligament), active (muscle) and control (coordination) systems.

This process of force detection and muscle reaction is the job of the control system. In some people this is very good and runs extremely smoothly. In a ballet dancer, for example, the muscles may be small and lean, but because body control is very good the dancer can use just the right amount of muscle force to hold the body stable and control each action with great precision. After a knee injury, a rugby player may still have much bigger muscles than the ballet dancer, but body control has been compromised by pain.

The muscles shake and quiver as the knee moves and actions are ungainly and poorly controlled.

In the case of the lumbar spine, which is clearly in the centre of the body (axial skeleton), the stability provided by the active, passive and control systems is of the 'core' of the body. In this case the active system is that of the abdominal and lumbar muscles, while the passive system consists of the spinal bones, discs and ligaments. The control system integrating these two comes from nervous impulses in both the spine and brain.

The muscles of the active sub-system can be divided into the surface (superficial) muscles of the rectus abdominis and the external obliques which primarily move the core region, and the deeper muscles, transversus abdominis and internal obliques, and multifidus which mainly prevent excessive movement of the body core and 'stabilise' it.

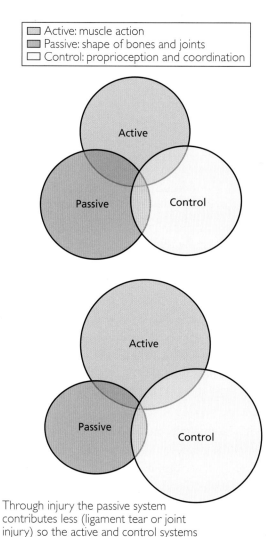

□ Active: muscle action
□ Passive: shape of bones and joints
□ Control: proprioception and coordination

Through injury the passive system contributes less (ligament tear or joint injury) so the active and control systems may be improved through rehabilitation to compensate

Figure 4.1 Stabilisation mechanisms of the lumbar spine

> **Key point**
> Muscles function not just to create movement, but to protect the body against excessive motion created from external forces acting upon it.

For effective core stability, a subtle interplay between the three systems is required. The bones and joints must move freely, the muscles must be strong and supple, and the body control must be well coordinated. Failure of any one of these systems will reduce core stability. Importantly, however, if this does occur, correctly applied exercise can often build up the other two stability components to compensate (see fig. 4.1). Take arthritis as an example. In this condition there is wear and tear on the joints. This can often leave the joint less stable with a tendency to give way. In this situation, a physiotherapist or personal trainer can give a patient rehab exercises to strengthen

Table 4.1	Stabilising muscles of the lumbar spine	
Muscle category	**Local**	**Global**
Anatomical position	• Closer to the spine	• More distant from the spine
Muscle name	• Multifidus • Transversus abdominis • Internal oblique • Quadratus lumborum (medial portion) • Psoas	• External oblique • Rectus abdominis • Quadratus lumborum (lateral portion) • Iliacus
Reaction to injury & pain	• Poorly recruited • Laxity • Waste	• Spasm & trigger point development • Can tighten • May thicken
Rehabilitation aim	• Enhance recruitment • Build endurance	• Release trigger points • Lengthen • Reduce dominance

the muscles that support the joint and improve the body control by using skilled movements. The active and control components of stability are therefore built up to compensate for the wear on the passive system. Although the bones cannot be changed, the patient enjoys almost full, pain-free actions because the body has compensated for the damaged joints and bones. The essential principle here is that full function can be restored, even when a structural detriment remains.

LOCAL AND GLOBAL MUSCLES

We saw in chapter 1 that we have two sets of muscles contributing to core stability. One set – the local muscles – is close to the central core of the body. The other set – the global muscles – is more distant from the central core. The local muscles, close to the spine and pelvis, act to move the spine subtly and adjust it with fine movements to keep posture correct and make sure that body alignment is optimal. One of the most important functions is to stiffen the spine. If you imagine the spine as a flexible column of individual bones, when it is subjected to forces from outside the body there will be a tendency for the column to bend. When the local muscles are contracted, it is as though tape has been wound around the column, making it stiffer.

The local muscles are switched on ('recruited') before the global muscles in many actions, a process termed pre-activation. The global muscles, on the other hand, do not make fine adjustments of spinal position, but instead take some of the strain that the body is subjected to before it can damage the spine. When lifting an object, for example, the large leg muscles attaching to the pelvis (global) can be used to provide the power for the lift while the deep muscle corset (local) can maintain the neutral position of the lower spine. The global muscles tend to be more involved in larger movements and especially rapid ballistic actions in sport.

Often, after a bout of back pain, the local muscles are turned off and quickly waste (become lax). Going further, the local muscles tend to be inhibited, hypotonic, have delayed activity, and demonstrate atrophy weakness.

In contrast to this, the global muscles tend to react to injury by becoming overactive, tight and short, and therefore come to dominate movements which then lose their subtle control. The tone of the muscles increases making them firmer to palpation, while the actin and myosin fibres move closer together effectively shortening the muscle. Because the muscle now has higher tone, when a movement requires several muscles to work the higher toned muscle has a tendency to switch on first (this is called 'preferential recruitment') and so comes to dominate the movement. Both muscle sets can react to stress and emotion: the global muscles by tightening and going into painful spasm, the local muscles by becoming hypotonic. A typical example of this would be tightness in the neck, jaw and upper trapezius muscles during bouts of anxiety or the reduction in tone of the shoulder retractor muscles allowing the shoulders to slump forwards in cases of depression.

In cases of instability, when we move we lose subtle movements of the spine and rely instead on our large global muscles. Our movements become clumsy and poorly coordinated, and the muscles often become tight, tense and painful. For example, after a bout of gardening, your back might feel stiff, with tight, cord-like muscles. Instead of using the subtle local musculature of the body core, we have used the strong global muscles. They are too powerful for this task,

Definitions of muscle changes

Inhibition is a process where impulses from another nerve (normally caused by pain or swelling) override the impulses that would otherwise instigate muscle contraction.

Hypotonia is lower than normal muscle tone so the muscle feels less firm at rest.

Delayed activity simply means that in a movement sequence the local muscles move slightly later than they should, often meaning that the movement has begun without a stable base being established first.

Atrophy weakness means that the muscle is weak because it has wasted and become physically smaller. This is normally a result of prolonged inactivity.

however, and quickly go into spasm, causing pain. If we make the mistake of trying to strengthen the back in a gym using heavy weight-training techniques, the already firm global muscles can be built up even further without an attendant increase in the local muscles, so we end up with an imbalance between the two sets of muscles, resulting in further pain.

The initial work of rehab in the clinic is to perform gentle foundation movements designed to restore muscle balance, and work to improve core stability by targeting the local muscles. Once these have been performed and core stability has been improved, the exercises gradually bring in the global muscles to build complete 'spinal fitness' in the gym.

THE ABDOMINAL BALLOON

If we look at the whole trunk we can imagine it as a cylinder, formed by the ribcage and abdomen (see fig. 4.2). This cylinder is divided across the centre by the diaphragm. In effect we have two cylinders, thoracic and abdominal, sharing a common ceiling and floor.

The walls of the upper part of the cylinder (thoracic) are formed by the ribcage and muscles attaching to it, while those of the lower cylinder (abdominal) are the oblique abdominal muscles which constitute the deep muscle corset (transversus, internal obliques and multifidus). The top of the abdominal cylinder and base of the thoracic cylinder is formed by the diaphragm, a sheet of muscle tissue, which 'cuts the body in half' and is found beneath the chest and above the abdomen. This muscle enables us to breathe, pulling air into the lungs and forcing it out again like a pair of bellows. When we breathe in, the diaphragm goes down to pull air into the lungs. Because it goes down, the top of the abdominal cylinder is squashed in, rather like pressing on the top of a drinks can. The floor of the cylinder is formed by the pelvic floor muscles (see chapter 1), the ones that help us hold on when we are desperate to go to the toilet but can't find the

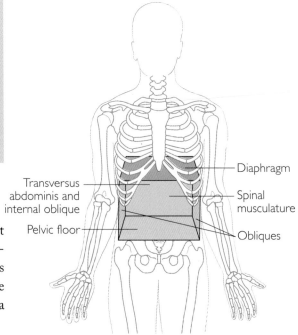

Figure 4.2 The abdominal balloon

bathroom! When we do this, these muscles are pulled into the body slightly giving us the feeling that we are pulling in and upwards between the legs.

When all three sets of muscles work together, the cylinder is squeezed in every direction: the top is pulling down, the bottom is pulling up and the walls are squeezing inwards. Contained within the cylinder are the stomach, intestines and bodily organs, and as the muscles squeeze in, the whole area acts like a giant balloon, providing a solid 'bubble' at the front of the trunk. As we lift a heavy object there is a tendency for the spine to buckle and bend forwards (flex), but the abdominal balloon – positioned at the front of the body – helps to stop this happening. This

Key point

The abdominal balloon is created by the abdominal muscles, pelvic floor muscles and diaphragm

mechanism of pressure within a cylinder works a little like the gas in a fizzy drink. When empty, the drinks can may be crushed easily but when full with the gas under pressure it becomes rigid. Pressure within the abdominal cylinder has a similar effect of support, reinforcing what is essentially a hollow vessel.

Heavy lifts or rapid movements of the trunk result in stronger muscle contractions and so the pressure produced by the abdominal balloon is greater. As this pressure is within the abdomen, it is called intra abdominal pressure, or IAP. Similarly when we take a deep breath into the lungs and expand the chest cavity, the increase in pressure within the chest is called intrathoracic pressure (ITP).

Intra thoracic pressure (ITP) is increased following a deep breath and can be maintained if the breath is held. The 'Valsalva manoeuvre', consisting of a deep breath, held against a closed glottis, may be performed in conjunction with an abdominal contraction. The Valsalva manoeuvre compresses the aorta and vena cava (which pass through the diaphragm) and increases blood pressure. Although a natural movement which occurs during strain activities, the increase in blood pressure makes the manoeuvre undesirable during rehabilitation. Valsalva may be used by the experienced weightlifter during activities such as the squat or dead lift action, but the period for which the breath is held should be brief.

The Valsalva manoeuvre will also increase IAP via movement of the diaphragm. When breathing in, the diaphragm is pulled downwards (or 'descended') and when breathing out, the diaphragm is pulled upwards (ascended). Higher levels of IAP are produced during inhalation and breath holding, a position that combines downward movement of the diaphragm with Valsalva.

Interestingly, because all three sets of muscles that form the abdominal cylinder have to tighten at the same time to increase IAP, the coordination of this action can break down. One example of this is the incontinence affecting some recent mothers. This occurs sometimes when they cough

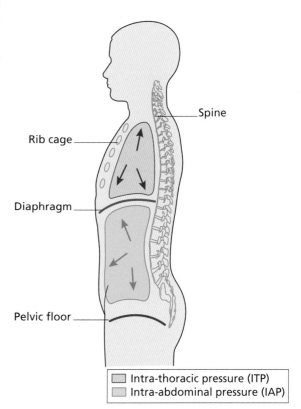

Figure 4.3 Intrathoracic pressure

or laugh because both of these actions increase IAP. Although the pressure is increasing, the pelvic-floor muscles are poorly toned and poorly controlled after pregnancy, so the pressure causes urine to press out of the bladder unrestrained. This problem can be solved by restoring the ability to feel the muscles between the legs are pulling 'in and up' by using special pelvic-floor exercises and also targeting the deep muscle corset.

The larger the IAP and ITP, the better a person's core stability – this is achieved by having deep abdominal muscles which are strong, but more importantly able to hold the area firm for long periods. This is why holding, or muscle endurance, is important to core stability.

Key point

Intra abdominal pressure (IAP) is the inward squeezing force created as the muscles forming the abdominal balloon tighten. Intra thoracic pressure (ITP) is the pressure created in the ribcage by taking a deep breath and holding it.

BACK FASCIA

The second method by which core stability is created involves a sheet of tough elastic membrane which stretches from the back of the ribcage to the pelvis. The material is called 'fascia' and because this particular piece stretches across the upper back (thoracic spine) and lower back (lumbar spine) it is called the 'thoraco-lumbar fascia' or TLF. As we lift an object and are pulled forwards by its weight, the fascia is stretched. However, several muscles work to pull on the fascia and tighten it, enabling it to resist this force because the transver-

sus abdominis and the internal oblique surround the trunk and attach to the fascia at the back, through a slightly thickened region called the lateral raphe. When these muscles tighten they pull the fascia from the sides, similar to the effect of pulling on the side of someone's shirt to flatten it.

The back muscles (spinal extensors) are two strong vertical columns running up either side of the spine. They are encased in a layer of the fascia, and when they contract they also stretch the fascia and tighten it. The effect of the spinal extensors is actually increased (by as much as 30 per cent, according to some calculations) by being enclosed by fascia, and this increase is called the hydraulic amplifier effect. This effect actually occurs with several muscle groups throughout the body. Cutting the fascial surrounding of a muscle (fasciotomy) significantly reduces the muscle power output.

Definition

A hydraulic amplifier effect occurs when a muscle expands and pushes outwards against the restriction of a surrounding elastic facial envelope, which pulls inwards. The effect is seen in a number of body areas including the spinal extensor muscles (thoracolumbar fascia) and vastus lateralis of the leg (fascia lata).

The buttock muscles (gluteals) and the muscles which pull your arms to your sides (latissimus dorsi) connect to the bottom and top of the TLF respectively. They tighten it by pulling the TLF downwards and upwards (longitudinal tension) at the same time as the deep abdominal muscles pull it sideways (transverse tension) see fig. 4.4.

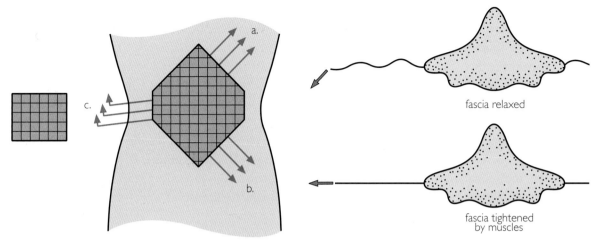

Figure 4.4 The back fascia (a) Latissimus dorsi (b) Gluteals (c) Transversus abdominis

The net result of all this muscular activity is to strengthen the spine and help it resist the bending forces inherent in lifting. They create an effective mechanism, but one which can only function optimally if the muscles are strong and able to pull for a long period of time. In addition, the muscles must work at the correct point in a lift. If they pull too soon their force will be worthless, and if they pull after the weight has been lifted, the stress will already have been placed on the spine. Again, coordination is important. The muscles must pull at just the right time, with just the right amount of force – and, after a bout of back pain or a long period of inactivity, this mechanism takes training and practice to restore.

Key point

The deep abdominals, gluteals, erector spinae and latissimus muscles all connect to the thoracolumbar fascia (TLF). By tightening it these muscles help stabilise the spine.

BREATHING MECHANISM

When we breathe, both the ribcage and abdominal wall move. During inspiration (breathing in) the diaphragm and external intercostal muscles contract to expand the ribcage and draw the diaphragm down, thereby increasing the volume of the chest cavity. As the depth and force of inspiration is increased, secondary muscles come into play, including the upper trapezius, pectoralis major and minor, sternocleidomastoid and scalene muscles. This is more marked if the upper limb is fixed, providing a stable base for the muscles to pull against. As inspiration deepens, the thoracic spine extends to flatten its contour through activity of the spinal extensors to facilitate a greater movement. The diaphragm also requires a stable base, and this is provided by the muscles that anchor the lower ribs and lumbar vertebrae, including the transversus, psoas, and quadratus lumborum.

During expiration (breathing out) the intercostal muscles relax and the passive recoil provides the force for quiet breathing. When expiration is forced, the deep abdominal muscles contract to depress the thoracic floor and deflate the rib cage to narrow the thoracic outlet. This hollowing action constricts the abdomen.

Three categories of breathing are commonly recognised: abdominal (or diaphragmatic), lower lateral costal and apical (upper chest). In abdominal breathing the diaphragm alone is active, with little chest movement during gentle breathing. This is generally thought to be the most efficient form of breathing, with the diaphragm doing up to 80 per cent of the work of inspiration at a cost of less than 5 per cent of the body's energy (Key, 2010). Lower lateral costal breathing occurs as the lower ribs flare out (the so-called 'bucket handle' movement of the rib cage). Apical breathing sees the ribs moving upwards and forwards in the so-called 'pump handle movement' of the rib cage. Apical breathing is the least efficient mechanism and is seen in strained hyperventilation, which can use as much as 30 per cent of body energy.

(a) Bucket handle

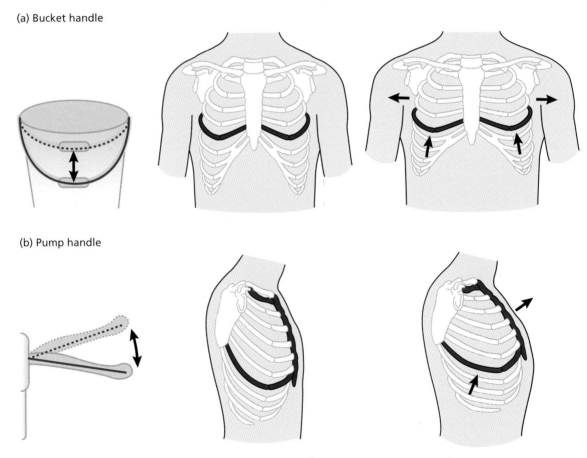

(b) Pump handle

Figure 4.5 Rib movement in breathing

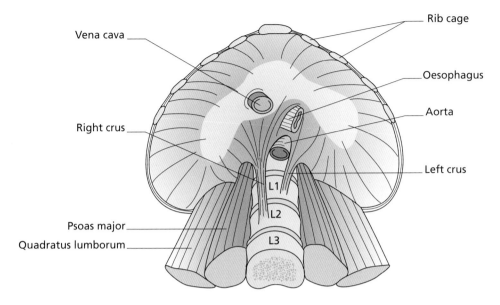

Figure 4.6 Structure of the diaphragm

During the respiratory cycle the spine and pelvis move sequentially. At the beginning of an in breath the sacrum moves and the respiratory wave passes up the spine to finish at the base of the neck. If the breath is held due to fright, the abdomen is braced and the movement of the chest and ribcage is blocked. The diaphragm cannot descend and intra-abdominal pressure increases. If this becomes habitual, breathing can be restricted to the apical regions alone, giving the appearance of a central belt tightened around the mid-body.

DIAPHRAGM IN RELATION TO STABILITY

The diaphragm is positioned between the abdomen and ribcage, a little like a mushroom. The mushroom stem is formed by the right and left crus, two muscular pillars attaching to the inner surface of the lumbar vertebrae and discs as an extension from the anterior longitudinal ligament of the spine. The right crus is longer and thicker than the left. The stem of the diaphragm is closer to the spine than to the front of the body, and the muscular fibres of the diaphragm edge are attached around the inner ribcage (inferior thoracic outlet), converging on a broad central tendon sheet. Muscular fibres of the diaphragm thus attach to the sternum, lumbar spine and ribcage. These attachments extend as high as the seventh rib and as low as L3. When the diaphragm contracts it will produce tension across its central tendon, to the base of the ribcage and the inner surface of the lumbar spine: it is this latter action which enables the diaphragm to contribute to the stability of the lumbar spine. The Crural region – formed by the right and left crus – pulls directly on the bodies of L2 and L3 and appears to lengthen the spine. Where the spine and lower ribs are stabilised the diaphragm will pull its dome down towards the pelvis as it contracts. This action will be checked by an increase in IAP, and represents abdominal breathing (see above). The descended diaphragm now rests on the abdominal organs, and the force of its contraction causes the ribs to lift and widen in the horizontal plane.

SENSORIMOTOR REHABILITATION

Normally when we train in a gym, we use specific exercises with individual aims such as strength or stretching, or targeted at specific body parts such as leg or arm exercises. This isolation approach, while effective, does not replicate the normal day-to-day activity of the body, and as such it can be criticised for being non-functional. Functional activities use whole-body movements which mimic day-to-day activities, or actions in daily work or sport. In so doing they use several body parts together to rehearse the coordination and muscle timing inherent in the relevant action. Sensorimotor rehabilitation couples the sensory (feeling) and motor (movement) systems, using the brain and central nervous system to provide a link between the two.

In reality all exercise is sensorimotoric to a certain extent as it is impossible to move without feeling the action. However, many standard gym

exercises do not focus on the quality of the movement. Users often find themselves distracted by music or a training partner and pay little attention to the sensory aspect of the exercise. Sensorimotor rehabilitation increases the emphasis of the feeling of the movement to enhance its quality.

Sensorimotor rehabilitation uses standard models of motor skill acquisition to improve coordination in exercise. Frequently, a developmental approach is used to reflect the way in which we put basic reflex-driven actions together to form motor programmes as we develop from babies through childhood to adults. These motor programmes form the basis of posture and locomotion and are therefore vital to models of back rehabilitation.

Sensorimotor training involves the use of proprioceptive input from joints and muscles, locomotor reflexes (these are involuntary modifications of movement, which help us, for example enabling us to walk from early childhood) and cerebellar activity from the part of the brain responsible for balance and coordination. Table 4.2 shows some types of activities commonly used.

In order to understand sensorimotor training we first need to look at the method by which people learn skilled movements (motor skills).

HOW CLIENTS LEARN SKILLED EXERCISE

We can think of the human organism a little like a modern machine such as a computer. Information is presented as an input (your instructions to your client), your client processes this information (deciding what to do and determining how to do it), before producing an output – in this case an exercise. Viewing actions in this way is called an 'information processing model' (see fig. 4.7). It is important to note that humans are not simply

> ### Key point
> Sensorimotor rehabilitation uses exercises that emphasise both the sensory (feeling) and motor (movement) systems.

Table 4.2	Sensorimotor training
Type	**Method**
Proprioception	Increase proprioceptive input through sole of foot, head position & major joints.
Postural stability	Challenge stability using variation of base of support and labile surfaces.
Motor programmes	Activate recovery strategies to use predetermined (ingrained) motor patterns.
Function	Use functional activities relevant to daily living, work and/or sport.

Source: Page, P., et al., *Assessment and treatment of muscle imbalance: the Janda approach* (Champaign, IL: Human Kinetics, 2010)

responding to the information which is taken in, but processing it. As we will see later this implies that there is an interaction between currently held information (knowledge) and new information (input) in order to produce a particular movement (output).

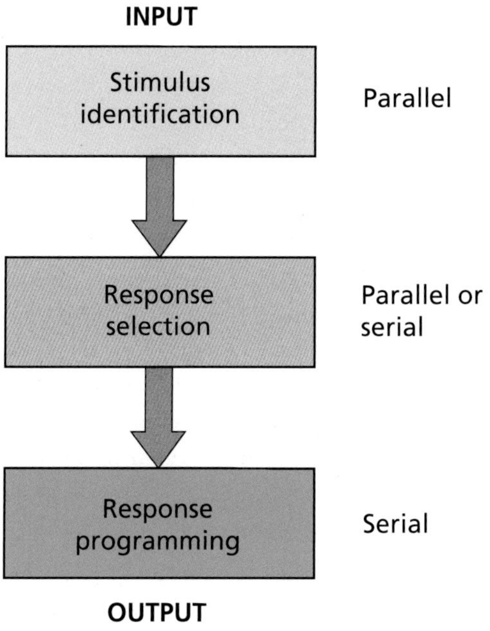

The first stage in this process is stimulus identification. Imagine that you are at a party and everyone is talking. You are capable of hearing each voice, but choose not to: they simply register as a general background din. Then, someone mentions your name and you look up – what has happened? Suddenly you have decided to tune into one sound rather than all the others. You have applied a technique called selective attention. This is your natural filter mechanism, which screens out things which you think are not important, picking up instead on things which you think are important.

It is quite possible for you to hear, see, feel, smell, and taste several things at once. Doing

INPUT

Stimulus identification — Parallel

Response selection — Parallel or serial

Response programming — Serial

OUTPUT

Figure 4.7 The information processing model

Definition

Selective attention is a cognitive psychology term for a person's ability to pick out one stimulus (for example sound) within a field of numerous stimuli.

this is called 'parallel processing', because it all happens at the same time. Once you have received a stimulus which demands a response (for example pain from stepping on a pin demands that you should move your foot to limit skin damage) you have started the process of 'response selection'. This stage can use either parallel processing or serial processing. 'Serial processing', as might be expected, involves performing actions one after another. In the response selection phase of information processing, actions at which we are well practised may be processed in parallel, while unfamiliar or complex actions require more thought and need to be practised in series. Once we have determined what response to make (we are going to move our foot off the pin) we need to programme the action in terms of coordination and muscle work. This process occurs in series and is termed 'response programming'.

At the response selection and response programming stages of the process there can be interaction with currently held knowledge. At the input stage, stimuli are detected and the interaction with current knowledge gives them meaning. So for example when you are walking in the country and you see movement on the ground some distance ahead you may perceive this as a rabbit. When you get to the spot of ground you see that it was really an empty crisp bag. The visual stimulus is the same in each case (the light reflecting from the bag into your eye) but the perception has changed. You perceived a rabbit because you compared the visual stimuli to memories of previous similar events and that was the one that seemed to match most closely.

At the response programming stage you are able to draw on stored movement programmes. These are individual movements that have been pieced together to produce a single sequence. So for example throwing a ball may consist of the individual movements: stepping (A), trunk twisting (B), shoulder movement (C), elbow movement (D), hand movement (E). The throwing action is a single programme which when begun runs A+B+C+D+E as a single sequence.

> **Definition**
>
> A motor programme is a series of neural commands which when initiated results in a single sequence of coordinated movements.

Importantly, from a rehab perspective, clients are often able to learn new actions if they are linked to familiar movements. For example, if we are trying to teach abdominal hollowing as part of a core training programme the action is quite difficult to understand for someone unfamiliar with exercise. Saying 'pull your tummy in as though you were trying to squeeze into a tight pair of jeans' links to a motor programme which the client is already familiar with rather than having to learn an entirely new muscle action.

Because several simple tasks can be processed in parallel while only one more complex task can be processed at a time, a bottleneck is created (see fig. 4.8). This means that a complex action must be completed before another action can be begun. As many new exercise actions are tricky for beginners, it is important to limit the number of movements learned. Failure to do this will result in the actions interfering with each other and becoming less effective. The answer is to keep things simple in the early stages of teaching an exercise. Once the client becomes more adept at performing an

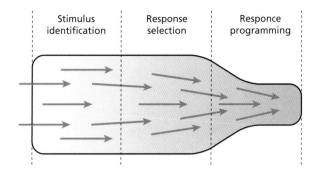

Stimulus identification | Response selection | Responce programming

Figure 4.8 Information processing bottleneck

action, it requires less attention and other actions may be introduced in parallel. Let's look at the practical application of the information processing model in exercise therapy by reviewing techniques of motor learning.

MOTOR LEARNING

Motor learning has been defined as a set of processes associated with practice or experience which leads to a relatively permanent change in the capability for skilled movement (Schmidt and Lee, 2011). The learning process itself cannot be directly observed because it occurs internally, but we can judge the effectiveness of the learning which has occurred by observing results. In other words we can monitor how the action has improved as a result of the teaching and learning we have given.

Motor learning is achieved through the three interrelated stages shown in table 4.3.

> ### Definition
> Motor learning is the process of learning skilled movements.

Table 4.3	Components of motor learning
Stage	**Practical application**
Cognitive (understanding)	• Use proper demonstration and cueing • Split complex actions into simpler subunits • Short bouts of exercise with precision • No home practice
Associative (effective movement)	• Link subunits together to form a single task • Less cueing required • Self-practice when client can identify own mistakes • Increase repetitions
Autonomous (automatic action)	• Reduce attention to task • Perform other actions while task is used • Increase task speed learning

Stage one

The first stage (cognitive) occurs when your client is finding out what is required of them, and for this reason the cognitive stage is often referred to as the stage of understanding. Here, your client is trying to form an idea of the whole movement. The process is very much 'thinking' (cognitive) rather than 'doing' (motor) in nature. If we take a hip hitch movement as an example (in which the client stands on a step with one leg hanging off it, and drops the unsupported leg to the ground, keeping both legs straight). This action may be very familiar to you, but to your client it is completely new. If you demonstrate the action quickly it will be difficult for them to work out what you are doing and what is required for successful performance of the exercise. If you are dressed in shorts so they can see the movement clearly, slow the action down, and point directly to your hip and pelvis and tell them that your pelvis is lifting and your leg is kept straight, the action becomes easier for them to understand. What you are really doing here is using environmental cues to facilitate their learning. As the client becomes more practised, these cues may no longer be necessary. The use of cues is explained below.

Your client is really working out how they can move their body to perform the action. We say that they are developing strategies to perform the end result (or goal). Sometimes these strategies will work and will be retained, and sometimes they won't and they will be lost.

Performance during the cognitive stage of motor learning will be poorly coordinated, and your client will need to pay close attention to what they are doing. Your client must concentrate intensely and will therefore become tired easily. You can assist them by providing clear instructions and feedback. Complex actions should be split up into more simple components. For example, a single leg hop and twist would first be learned as a single leg balance. Once your client is able to do this, you can progress to straight line hopping, followed by hopping and twisting on the spot and finally hopping and twisting over a distance. The aim is to split the action into manageable chunks of information. Some clients who are unfamiliar with exercise will need movements split up into more chunks and will need to spend longer learning each. Clients who regularly participate in sports will learn skills more quickly and will not need the task to be split up into as many separate components. We will look at part-task and whole-task training in more detail when we cover movement complexity later in this chapter.

Demonstration of the movement is important, and your client will need constant instruction and correction (i.e. coaching) to prevent them practising in the wrong way. It is very important to bear in mind that at the cognitive stage of learning your client may not be able to identify their own mistakes, so home exercise is inappropriate.

One of the ways we can help learning in this stage is to use *cueing*, to paint a mental picture of an action in terms that are easy to understand. A sensory cue is really a way of communicating with your client other than by simply giving instructions. For example, an abdominal hollowing action may be cued by asking the athlete to pull the tummy button in (a verbal cue) and showing them how to do it on yourself (a visual cue). You could use the clients own fingers to feel their abdomen tightening (a tactile, or 'haptic', cue). You can also use the intonation of your voice as you give instructions (an auditory, or verbal, cue) to indicate the intensity of the movement, and how long it should be held for. With many exercises we can use several cues: a process called multisensory cueing. For example, when lifting a heavy weight during bodybuilding, athletes will often shout at each other (auditory), gesticulate (visual) and even strike each other (tactile) to encourage greater performance. A similar process of multisensory

Definition

A cue is a signal that facilitates a particular action. Cues may be verbal, visual, auditory or tactile in nature. When a number of cues are used, the approach is termed 'multisensory'.

cueing is used by physiotherapists in the rehabilitation of neurological conditions.

Often when teaching an action to a client who rarely exercises it is important simply to get them to recognise or 'own' the part of their body which is affected. It may seem strange, but inactive individuals may not know, for example, that their abdomen can be pulled in, and will have little chance of learning this action quickly. This, combined with the fact that they are in pain means that we need to give them as much information as possible to be able to regain control of their body so that they may participate in the rehabilitation process. One of the ways we can do this is to make them identify more easily with a body part by focusing their attention on something which is familiar to them. For example rather than saying 'tighten your abdominal muscles' or 'pull your abdomen in' (both of which assume that your client knows where these areas are) we say 'pull your tummy button in'. In coaching terms this is encouraging them to better develop internal focus (their body) rather than their external focus (the environment).

Stage two

The second stage of motor learning is the associative stage, which is really the stage of effective movement. Here, your client will try to perform an exercise with more precision by refining it. It is as though the original clumsy action is 'whittled down' to a smoother defined movement. Importantly, through practice, your client is now able to recognise their own mistakes, and so self-practice (unsupervised home exercise) can now be useful. Their previous dependence on external cues such as visual and verbal encouragement from you now gradually gives way to being able to rely on their own feeling for when the movement is right. This type of feeling comes from proprioception (the ability to feel the quality of movement of the body), and is internal to them. Each time they perform a movement, their body will give them feedback about how well they performed; this information can be used to modify their next repetition of the exercise. Movements become more consistent, and your client is now able to work on the finer details of an action. Because the exercise is becoming more refined and efficient, it is less demanding both physically and mentally and so your client will be able to perform more repetitions. Greater repetition enhances performance still further.

The individual movement sequences that we used in stage one have now been linked together to give a longer skill sequence. The actions must still be slow and precise, with progression made only when the movement sequence is correct. Practising an incorrect action can still cause the movement to degrade, but by now the client should have a better idea of what constitutes a correct action.

Stage three

The third and final stage of motor learning is the autonomous stage, where the action seems to run by itself. This stage is often called 'automatic' (or 'grooved' in sporting circles). Because the action is so rapid, there is no time for feedback and instead the client must predict how they will perform an exercise by drawing on their previous learning. This type of performance is called *feedforwards*.

At this stage correct movements demand less attention, so your client will be able to perform other actions at the same time. By focusing on other actions, we are increasing the emphasis on automatisation of the original skill. For example, during ankle rehabilitation we may begin with ankle restrengthening and progress to a wobble board. Initially your client has to focus on keeping the edge of the board away from the floor while maintaining their own balance (cognitive stage). With repetition their ankle becomes stronger, their balance improves and they are able to perform the task (associative stage). Now, we can ask them to stand on the wobble board facing a wall and to throw and catch a basketball against the wall. Because their focus is on not dropping the ball, rather than remaining on the board, the balance and ankle stability becomes more automatic.

WHAT IS FUNCTIONAL TRAINING?

There is much talk within the field of rehabilitation about functional training, and this goes hand in hand with the sensorimotor approach highlighted above. Functional training aims to use exercises which replicate day-to-day activities as closely as possible. This contrasts sharply with traditional exercise, which often uses movements which exist in the gym alone. In general, functional movements are whole-body actions involving several joints and muscle groups at the same time. Because of this the amount of coordination and skill required is much higher. If we take as an example a leg extension movement, using a machine in the gym involves sitting in a chair with the shin pressed against a weight. The action is to straighten the knee to work the quadriceps muscles in isolation. For rehabilitation, this movement does have its uses following injury. For example, where the quadriceps muscles are working poorly, isolation can help to get them working. However, in a healthy, uninjured individual, training on a leg extension machine simply strengthens muscle without rehearsing normal movements. For this reason, we can categorise the leg extension machine as a non-functional action. In contrast, a step-up action involves movement at the ankle, knee, hip and lower spine. The quadriceps muscles are still used as with the leg extension, but now the stepping action is one used throughout the day (for example, when climbing the stairs). In addition, the quadriceps muscles are working in tandem with the hip extensors, calf muscles and upper body. Because this action mimics a day-to-day movement the exercise can be categorised as a functional movement.

Functional movements can constitute either an open or a closed kinetic chain. A kinetic chain is a sequence of moving elements. An example relevant to the human body is the bone components making up a limb. For example the leg is a kinetic chain made up of the foot, shin, and thigh bones. An open chain action is one where the end of the limb (hand for the upper limb, foot for the lower limb) moves freely. The proximal end of the limb (i.e. the end closest to the body) is fixed, while the distal end (i.e. the end most distant from the body) moves. This type of action is used in rapid movement such as throwing or the forward limb movement of running. A closed chain movement occurs when both ends of the limb are fixed. For example in a bench press action the proximal end of the arm remains on the bench while the distal end moves slowly with the bar. Another example is a squat where the foot is fixed on the floor and the hip moves slowly with the weight of the body. Open chain examples of these two exercises include an action such as dumbbell punching, where the hand moves rapidly, or kicking using a band resistance, where the foot moves rapidly. In both cases the rapid and relatively unhindered movement of the end of the limb categorises the action as open chain. Open chain actions are often rapid movements such as punching and kicking where the limb can move in a ballistic action. Here, muscles begin and end the movement, but the middle part of the action also relies on the momentum of the moving limb. You are literally throwing the limb into the action. This requires large acceleration and deceleration forces at the beginning and end of the action, and the muscle work involved is very subtly coordinated. During the final stages of rehabilitation, the type of coordination required for ballistic actions is particularly important to retrain. Ballistic actions are used functionally in sport, but are less easy to spot in work and day-to-day actions. For example, a rhythmic gardening activity is ballistic in nature, as is swinging a child in your arms.

Closed chain actions are generally slower movements requiring co-contraction of muscles, that is muscles on either side of the joint (these are known as the 'agonist' and 'antagonist' muscles) working together. In closed chain actions the joint is loaded (compressed) and the muscle works to stabilise the joint. During rehabilitation it is important to identify which actions are functional.

In addition, because closed chain actions favour stability and open chain actions favour mobility, it is appropriate to select a starting position which favours the required result. For example, a squatting action may be used to stabilise the knee and a leg extension action to build muscle speed.

The complexity of an exercise is important for coordination during functional actions. Initial actions should be relatively simple to understand, control and correct. Gradually, as confidence is gained, more complex actions can be employed. Where a movement is complex it can be divided into several component movements. Each individual movement can be practised and mastered before the components are put together. This type is called *part task* training, and is a useful method for rehabilitation of individuals who are not skilled in movement production. A disadvantage of this approach, however, is that fitting components together does not always result in a smooth single action. Another method is *whole task* training. Here the complex action is used and you accept that initially the performance of the action will be poor. Gradually the action improves as the various components of it are corrected. The analogy here is of creating a statue. Part task training builds it from blocks or bricks one at a time, whole task training begins with a solid block of stone, chipping away to reveal the whole statue.

The type of muscle work used during functional training is also important. Isometric actions are used to hold a joint firm and prevent excessive motion. They are the stabilising actions that protect a joint and are used extensively in core training. Building up the amount of time that a client can maintain an isometric contraction (holding time) is often important when re-educating stability following injury. For example, when treating low back pain we often target the deeper abdominal muscles using a drawing-in movement of the abdominal wall (hollowing) rather than a sit-up movement. Initially clients may find this hard to achieve, but eventually they will perceive a mild contraction. To progress this, rather than asking them to contract their muscles harder, we build holding time by asking them to perform the hollowing action for 3–5 secs, then 10-20 secs and finally 60-120 secs.

Eccentric actions are important because they often represent periods when the muscle is controlling movement of a joint when the body is lowering and decelerating. It is during these movements that joints often give way, and training eccentric actions will help to prevent this and give the client confidence. As an example, someone with knee pain often finds it far easier to go upstairs than to come down. Coming down is an eccentric action and each step takes longer than going up. We can train this action by progressing the lowering action using a step down from a shallow step (e.g. by standing on a book) then a larger step (wooden yoga brick) and finally a single stair.

Concentric actions are often the hardest to retrain when a muscle is very weak and this can be a source of considerable demotivation for clients. To retrain the actions begin with eccentric actions and follow with assisted concentric actions. For example, following a knee injury where a client finds it difficult to straighten their leg in a sitting position (sitting leg extension above), straighten their leg for them and then ask them to lower it slowly, building up the time of lowering (3 secs, 5 secs, 10 secs). Next, ask them to lift the upper leg while you support the lower leg to take some of its weight. Gradually ease off your lifting pressure as they become able to support more of their own limb weight. Here we are using the non-functional isolation action to establish a good physiological base upon which to build functional training at a later date.

BIOPSYCHOSOCIAL FACTORS IN LOW BACK PAIN

Traditional approaches to back pain focus very much on structural problems and aim to diagnose physical faults. This is a biomedical model and assumes that our client's symptoms are the result of a problem with the body's biology. This traditional model views back pain as somatic (caused by the body), and psychogenic aspects (those caused by the mind) are interpreted as secondary and often viewed negatively as though aspects of the client's condition are not real.

Although the incidence of low back pain (i.e. the number of people with the condition) has remained relatively stable during the twentieth century, there has been a dramatic increase in the amount of disability which this condition causes (see Waddell, 1987). This seemingly contradictory scenario indicates that a factor besides the physical condition of low back pain is causing the increase in disability. Using a biopsychosocial approach focuses on the interaction between biology (body structure), psychology (mental influences) and social influences (environmental factors). It has been calculated that approximately 80 per cent of back pain clients have a condition that is not based on damage to individual body structures; this is called non-specific low back pain. This type of condition is said to involve several elements as depicted in figure 4.9.

It is important to appreciate the distinction between disability and structure. Studies have shown that 65 per cent of individuals over the age of 50 show abnormalities of the lumbar spine when x-rayed, whether they experience pain or not, and 33 per cent show disc abnormalities on MRI. In addition 20 per cent of normal individuals under the age of 60 have herniated disks, which they are frequently unaware of (Accident Compensation Corporation, 2004).

> **Key point**
>
> With chronic low back pain there is a distinction between disability (how the client copes with day-to-day activities) and structure (pathological changes in the spine).

One of the essential tenets of the biopsychosocial model is that pain should not be the central focus of attention with low back pain. Decreasing pain will only reduce disability if the client is encouraged to return to their pre-injury activity levels as soon as possible. It is the clients reaction to the pain which is the important aspect. This reaction is often based on their understanding of pain and their emotional response to it. This in turn rests on the client's belief system and the social network in which they exist. Interestingly, psychosocial factors are more accurate at determining the likely outcome of back pain and its recurrence than physical tests. A client's belief system about pain is very important. An indi-

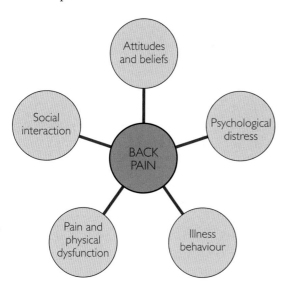

Figure 4.9 Biopsychosocial model of non-specific low back pain

vidual who equates pain with injury (hurt with harm) may have a very pessimistic view of their treatment progress, and be relatively noncompliant with a rehabilitation programme. They may fear an increase of their pain levels and therefore be less likely to fully commit to an exercise programme. In addition, the degree to which an individual believes they are in control of their pain can be a deciding factor in the eventual outcome of any treatment. The reliance on medical treatment takes the responsibility for recovery away from the individual, while the use of exercise places it firmly within their grasp. In this instance exercise can be used to empower the client and make them more self-reliant.

Definition

Acute low back problems (LBP) last for less than three months, recurrent LBP lasts less than three months but consist of episodes of acute LBP, chronic LBP lasts for more than three months.

Key point

During the management of lower back pain, exercise can be used to empower a client and increase self-reliance.

Western healthcare is largely based on a disease model, which assumes that pain is a result of tissue injury and that there is a logical progression from pain through to impairment and finally disability. It is generally believed that back pain involves the spine and nerves, is caused by an injury and is an irritable condition. These beliefs focus attention on single body parts and tissues rather than the whole person. The history and epidemiology of common low back pain shows us that back pain is actually an everyday symptom, and we are often unable to accurately identify any structural problem that can categorically be said to relate to all the patient's symptoms. Although we must recognise that back pain has its roots

in a physical problem, we must also be aware that some patients move on from this to develop chronic pain and disability, while others with the same level of tissue damage do not. Many individuals respond differently to the same type of back pain, and it is recognised within the field of medical research that social issues have a powerful influence on the behaviour of the condition. Pain and disability are not the same. Pain may be said to be a complex sensory and emotional experience, while disability is largely recognised as restriction to activity.

The key elements of the biopsychosocial model are shown in figure 4.9. This model argues that while back pain is a real physical problem, the dysfunction that it causes can vary tremendously between individuals. We constantly receive physical sensations about posture and movement and actively screen these (selective attention) so as not to overload the cognitive system. Any symptom that we perceive against this normal background has to be interpreted. The interpretation of a symptom as pain can be dependent on several coexisting factors. Beliefs and coping mechanisms are important to this process, as an inherent belief that a symptom is a threat to the body will lead to the symptom being interpreted as pain. Lets take the simple example of an exercise workout in the gym: an increased sensation within a body part or muscle would be interpreted positively as a sign of a good workout. That same intense sensation would be interpreted negatively if it is associated with a perceived injury, whether it be a muscle tear, disease state or chronic low back pain. Importantly, the sensation itself is the same in both cases, and it is only the interpretation that has changed. The anticipation of pain can often be far more limiting than pain itself. The belief that pain indicates disease or tissue damage (i.e. 'hurt equals harm') often causes an individual to avoid an action. In addition, it is common for clients to catastrophise – to believe that something is far worse than it actually is.

> **Definition**
>
> Catastrophising is 'thinking the worst' or 'looking on the dark side'. It can restrict thinking and force the client to focus on things which went wrong, rather than recognising that some things also went right.

It is important to differentiate between those who confront their pain and those who choose to avoid it. Pain confronters (those with an 'adaptive response') continue to be active, using activity as a distraction and a coping mechanism for their pain. In opposition to this, pain avoiders (those with a 'non-adaptive response') choose not to engage in activity, which clearly acts as a barrier to their long-term recovery, and makes them non-compliant with rehabilitation. These polar responses are part of a fear avoidance model (see Buer and Linton, 2002).

In the presence of distress, the severity of pain is often increased and pain tolerance may be significantly lowered. Anxiety, fear, depression and uncertainty may all increase our perception of bodily sensations.

In other mammals (and indeed in primitive man) sickness behaviour is used to enforce rest. Such traits as lethargy, sleepiness and depression ensure that the animal will rest to aid recovery. In modern man these factors are often exaggerated and extended and are termed illness behaviour. Illness behaviour refers to the use of descriptions that constantly focus on a client's condition rather than being neutral. An example of illness behaviour would be the continual use of a walking aid even when a leg injury has recovered, or continuing to rest when back pain is no longer present. Often, the client will develop a fear-avoidance belief, assuming that an activity will cause an injury or exacerbation of their condition. Unfortunately, healthcare individuals can reinforce this belief (the iatrogenic effect), by using misguided descriptions. Telling a client that they have 'curvature of the spine', a 'postural abnormality' or 'wear and tear', gives credence to a belief that there is a permanent physical change rather than a temporary effect. This type of description greatly rein-

> **Definition**
>
> Fear avoidance (fear of movement) is a process by which a client avoids certain activities based on fear and thus develops a disability. Illness behaviour consists of a set of adaptive changes that occur as the result of sickness, such as anxiety, lethargy, depression, loss of appetite, sleepiness and hyperalgesia. In other mammals they aid survival by enforcing rest, but are often exaggerated in humans.

forces the structure-orientated beliefs common in the biomedical model.

The social context in which back pain is experienced is also important. Family, work colleagues, and social networks can all influence clients' beliefs and coping strategies. Job satisfaction, litigation and compensation can all affect reporting of back pain, pain behaviour and recovery. The compensation-disability system can have a significant effect on recovery rate and has been found to be a strong predictor of return to work. Where an individual has to prove he or she is disabled to receive a financial benefit, it is less likely that a rehabilitation programme which reduces this disability and therefore potential payment will be effective. The social context also has important connotations for the healthcare provider as well. Failure to allow a return to work until an individual is fully pain-free for example can limit recovery and damage an individual's self-esteem.

EVALUATION AND INTERVENTION FOR PSYCHOSOCIAL FACTORS

To identify the existence of psychosocial factors in clients with low back pain it is necessary to listen to your client carefully. Observe their behaviour and body language and pay particular attention to both what is said and how your client says it. Try to empathise and understand what your client is feeling. Encourage them to talk about their fears in relation to back pain, offer both reassurance and correct any misunderstandings they may have concerning their clinical condition. In addition, expand the subjective examination to include your client's family, work and economic circumstances. The process of management of the psychosocial factors begins during the subjec-

tive examination itself. Identify negative beliefs and emotions and encourage positive thinking with the aim of changing a client's behavioural response to pain. In the rehabilitation programme pick achievable goals that build confidence and encourage a sense of control.

Identification of fear-avoidance patterns may also be carried out using standard questionnaires. The back behaviour questionnaire (BBQ) (Symonds *et al*, 1996) and the fear avoidance back questionnaire (FABQ) (Waddell *et al*, 1993) are two of the most common questionnaires used.

Psychosocial factors may be targeted using cognitive behavioural therapy (CBT) and computerised versions of this approach. In a study looking at self-management skills for chronic low back pain those who undertook a programme of guided relaxation and positive thinking fared better than a control group on all measured outcomes. The *Wellness Workbook* is available at iTunes, as a free download at the time of writing.

Psychological intervention in the clinical management of low back pain

* Listen to what is said and how your client says it (body language, facial expression, tone of voice);
* offer reassurance and correct misunderstandings about their condition;
* understand the client's family, work, and economic circumstances;
* identify negative beliefs and emotions;
* encourage positive thinking and relaxation;
* pick achievable goals during rehabilitation;
* build confidence and reinforce progress;
* encourage self-control.

CLIENT ASSESSMENT AND REHABILITATION PLANNING 5

Before designing an exercise for a client with low back pain it is essential to fully evaluate them both physically and clinically. If you are a therapist and do not have knowledge of exercise you will need to work with a personal trainer. Likewise if you are a trainer without clinical knowledge you should work with a therapist. Both aspects are important to correct rehabilitation.

RED FLAGS AND CONTRAINDICATIONS TO REHABILITATION

During client assessment a lot of information is available to us. We talk to our clients during our consultation, taking a history of their condition, ask questions and listen to the replies (subjective assessment). We examine movements, tissues and function (objective assessment). We then use this information to make an assessment of the client's condition and plan a rehabilitation programme. Through our evaluation, we have access to a variety of findings and have to determine how important each of these is. To make this task easier, we can highlight certain findings, which are more important than others. We use a process of flags, which highlight findings, and

may require referral for further investigation or close monitoring. Red flags are physical in nature and refer to findings that may indicate a more serious medical problem (pathology). Items such as infection, fracture or the presence of a tumour fall into this category. Yellow flags are psychosocial and indicate a psychological (mind) or social (environmental) issue that may be influencing the condition and have a bearing on the progress of rehabilitation.

> ### Key point
> Red flags are physical findings which may suggest a more serious condition underlying a client's back pain. Yellow flags are psychosocial factors, which may influence a client's recovery.

The first process we need to go through when examining a client with low back pain is diagnostic triage. This process categorises low back pain into one of three types: simple back pain, nerve root pain and possible serious pathology. The primary aim of diagnostic triage is to exclude serious pathology. Simple low back pain, which occurs within the 20 to 55 age group, shows pain that is mechanical in nature (meaning it is affected by a client's movements) and restricted to the lumbo-sacral or buttock area. It is categorised as low risk where the patient is generally medically well. Nerve root pain presents as unilateral symptoms, with pain intensity in the leg generally being greater than that in the lower back. Pain can radiate to the foot, giving altered sensation (paraesthesia), numbness and localised neurological deficit, such as reduction in reflexes or skin sensation, or muscle weakness for example.

Definition

A neurological deficit is an abnormality of a body part due to altered function of the brain, spinal cord or nerves. Examples in the low back include decreased sensation, weakness, altered walking pattern, balance problems, abnormal reflexes (increased or decreased), and loss of bladder or bowel control.

Straight leg raise (SLR) testing (see p. 98) generally reproduces pain, as this position stretches the sciatic nerve, which travels along the back of the thigh from the lower back. If something compresses this nerve or alters its conduction of electrical impulses, stretching the nerve using the SLR test reproduces the client's symptoms.

Possible serious spinal pathology can exist where there is evidence of red flags, especially in clients younger than 20 or older than 55, where pain is non-mechanical in nature (i.e. not influenced by movement) or where there is a history of cancer, prolonged steroid or drug use, or HIV. Marked structural deformity may also be present and the patient may be generally unwell (suffering weight loss, for example). Severe early-morning stiffness and thoracic pain should also be noted. Table 5.1 lists red flags. Where red flags are present, clients should be referred to a medical practitioner for further investigation.

As we saw in chapter 4, back pain may also be affected by psychological factors indicated by

Table 5.1	Red flags are clinical indicators of possible serious conditions requiring further medical examination and/or investigation	
Fracture	**Infection or tumour**	**Neurological deficit**
• Major trauma such as severe fall or traffic accident • Minor trauma as above in elderly or infirm	• Client aged over 50 or under 20 years • History of previous cancer • Systemic/constitutional symptoms such as fever or prolonged weight loss • Recent bacterial infection • Intravenous drug usage • Immunosuppression • Pain worse at night or when lying down	• Severe or progressive alteration in sensation (sensory nerve) or weakness (motor nerve) • Bladder or bowel dysfunction • Evidence of neurological deficit in legs or perineum

Table 5.2	Yellow flags are indicators of psychosocial influences which may influence a client's recovery

Belief that pain and activity is harmful or severely disabling (equating hurt with harm).

Avoiding an activity through fear that it will be painful (fear-avoidance behaviour).

Low or negative mood state and withdrawal from social networks (peers/work/family).

Expectation that only passive treatment (medication/hands on techniques) rather than active participation (activity or exercise therapy) will help.

Ongoing compensation claim or litigation.

Heavy workload, unsociable hours, poor job satisfaction.

Over-protective family or lack of support.

the presence of yellow flags. These are potential psychosocial barriers to recovery, such as the belief that pain is harmful (correlation between hurt and harm), fear-avoidance behaviour (avoiding a movement without trying it because you think it will hurt), and depression or low mood state. The belief that passive treatments such as medication, rather than active treatment such as rehabilitation is the only possible course of intervention is also classified as a yellow flag, as is the presence of a compensation claim. Table 5.2 indicates yellow flags.

CLINICAL REASONING

Clinical reasoning is a methodical approach used by therapists of all types to decide which treatments are appropriate, when they should be used and why. Rather than applying a standard treatment programme and using the same techniques with each client, we should assess our clients to determine their individual needs, and tailor their programme accordingly. Clinical reasoning (CR) is the thinking process that we go through during the evaluation and application of back rehabilitation. Through interaction with our clients, we gather information and use this to develop a *hypothesis* about what could be wrong and what we should do to help.

The process of CR involves interaction with our clients. When we do this we are really looking at them through a lens made up by our past knowledge and beliefs. Clearly the way that you look at a client as a qualified therapist or trainer will be very different to the way you would have

Definition

In clinical reasoning a hypothesis is a theory which could explain our client's symptom behaviour.

Table 5.3	The four key components to clinical reasoning
Beliefs What are your beliefs about injury and healing, and how do these influence your treatment choices?	**Hypothesis** What condition do you think explains your client's symptoms?
Assessment What information do you get from the client prior to, during and after treatment?	**Expertise** What clinical experience do you have of this particular condition?

looked before you entered your profession. CR involves four essential components (see table 5.3). CR entails collecting data (signs and symptoms), analysing this data (making decisions) and developing a treatment plan. It is important that you are able to justify why you are using a particular technique. What effect are you aiming at, and how will the back rehabilitation programme you design affect your client's condition?

How do we gain the information we need? Basically there are five ways in which clinical information is gained or influenced. Where we think the client's symptoms are coming from (the source), what makes their symptoms better or worse (contributing factors), what we should be cautious of when examining the client or prescribing rehab (precautions), how we are going to intervene (management), and how we think they will react to our intervention (prognosis).

SOURCE

As soon as your client walks into the room, you are assessing them. How they walk, talk and move will all give clues. Contrast your view of someone who bounces into the room, bends over effortlessly to kick off their shoes and tells you they have just come back from a five-mile run, with

someone who walks in slowly showing pain on their face and is unable to bend or reach forwards. The former client is less likely to have chronic low back pain than the latter. You have no proof of this of course, but your hypothesis is that because one client has unlimited movement, while the other reacts in a way that you have seen in those with back pain. The essential feature here is that you have received information and compared it to your previous experience. Clearly, the experienced practitioner will be able to do this far better than a student, so the level of expertise that you have in relation to a clinical condition will influence your choice of treatment.

At the end of your assessment you will have made a decision about the source of your client's symptoms, and as you go through your assessment and gain further information you will support or disprove this hypothesis.

By continuing to gather information and compare it to what you think is wrong with your

Key point

Your expertise in relation to a clinical condition will influence your choice of treatment.

client you are reviewing your hypothesis. Sometimes the information may support your hypothesis. If you think your client has back pain when they come into the room, the fact that they experience pain when they bend to untie their shoes would support this. If they can bend freely and are able to get onto the couch easily, your original hypothesis of severe back pain may be incorrect.

Key point

As treatment progresses, you gain further information from your client and apply the process of reflection to support, modify or refute your hypothesis.

CONTRIBUTING FACTORS

Contributing factors are those that aggravate your client's condition. These can sometimes be more important than the source of the problem itself. For example the source of the problem may be your client's back muscles (erector spinae) and the contributing factor could be repeated bending at work. Clearly unless you give your client advice about good back care and avoiding bending, their condition will not improve.

PRECAUTIONS

Precautions to evaluation and treatment are things that don't allow your client's condition to settle (repeated bending in the above example) or make it worse because they continue to stretch the tissues. These are important as you will need to identify anything which stirs your client's condition up to avoid exacerbating it. If, for example, a client has an inflamed tendon which is made worse by mild movement, it would be unwise to use a vigorous treatment technique or exercise. The fact that mild movement has made it worse would suggest that excessive movement should be avoided.

MANAGEMENT

In deciding how to manage a client's condition, you must decide whether or not exercise therapy is appropriate. It is easy to assume that the very fact that a client has come to see you means they are in need of treatment. It is important, however, to be able to say that a particular treatment technique is inappropriate at this stage and to be willing to refer the client on to another healthcare provider or medical practitioner.

PROGNOSIS

If you are satisfied that strength training (for example) is appropriate you must now decide which techniques should be used and why (i.e. you must undertake justification of your technique). As treatment progresses, you will gain continual feedback from your client: what they feel, how their body reacts to treatment and how they feel after treatment. These factors will give you an idea about the likely outcome following treatment (prognosis) and enable you to prepare your client for this. For example, is it likely that a client who has suffered from knee pain for six months will be pain-free after a single treatment? They may expect to be, but your clinical experience with other patients and the nature of the healing process will suggest that several treatment sessions will be required. Remember also that therapy cannot cure everything. Clients will often put pressure on you to get them better, but in some cases a condition may be too serious or have progressed too far for you to realistically be able to help.

CLIENT EVALUATION

How do we gain information from our client to enable us to come up with a hypothesis to explain their complaint? Evaluation is most easily structured using the mnemonic SOAP, standing for Subjective, Objective, Assessment and Plan (see fig. 5.1).

SUBJECTIVE ASSESSMENT

Making a subjective assessment involves questioning your client, or taking a history, and we have begun this process by looking at red and yellow flags above. Clinical conditions often have a definite pattern, for example an acute injury (one which happens suddenly) would normally indicate a historical injury (for example, a twist or strain), while a chronic injury (one that develops slowly) will usually have resulted from overuse of a body part during a regular activity such as sport.

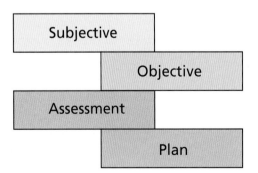

Figure 5.1 The SOAP chart is helpful for assessing your client's needs

Table 5.4	These are the categories you should typically question during your subjective assessment
Category	
Age and occupation	
Site and spread	
Onset and duration	
Symptoms and behaviour	
Medical considerations	

Now, by extending our subjective assessment we aim to identify these patterns. To do this we should ask questions in a variety of categories and as a guide table 5.4 shows typical categories used by physiotherapists in this respect.

Age and occupation

These are important, because certain conditions, such are osteoarthritis, are more common in older clients. Low back pain can occur in anyone, but manual workers have very different stresses imposed on the spine than desk-bound individuals, for example. In addition the advice for aftercare will obviously vary, so gaining a wider knowledge of the typical activities to which a client is returning is important.

Site and spread

The site and spread of symptoms (something a client complains of) can give clues to pain referral. For example a disc injury in the low back may trap the sciatic nerve sending pain into the leg (known as 'sciatica'). Sometimes a client may complain of leg pain and be unaware that they have a back condition. Equally, pain can be referred from a condition even when a nerve is not trapped. For example a frozen shoulder may often cause a deep gnawing pain, which travels across the front of the shoulder and into the upper arm. Failure to identify this could lead to treatment of the wrong tissues, targeting the arm rather than the shoulder itself.

Onset and duration

Asking about the onset of symptoms will clarify the difference between a sudden onset (acute) condition and that which develops slowly over time (overuse), and will help you to identify the stage of healing and the likely condition of the injured tissues.

Symptoms and behaviour

Learning more about symptoms and their behaviour will give you information about things which make the client's condition better or worse. For example, a chronic stiff joint is typically improved by gentle mobilising exercise, while an acute joint normally reacts to exercise with increasing pain as the condition is stirred up; this is something you would need to avoid in a treatment plan.

Medical considerations

A medical history should be taken, as it is important to know if a client has medical conditions beyond the injury they are presenting you with and whether or not they are taking any medication which may affect or be affected by rehabilitation. A simple medical questionnaire should be filled in prior to treatment, and you should question your client more closely on areas which are likely to be affected by rehab. Always liaise with your client's GP to ensure that your treatment does not conflict with treatments being given by other practitioners.

OBJECTIVE ASSESSMENT

Objective assessment is your physical evaluation of the client, and for the lumbar spine we can structure the process into a broad screening evaluation and more specific special tests, the latter being more relevant to the clinic than to the gym. Physical evaluation uses a mixture of active, passive and resisted movements.

Definition

Active movements are those performed by the client, passive movements are performed by the therapist on the client and resisted movements use isometric muscle contraction with the client's joints remaining still.

Active movements show the quality of movement and the body's willingness to move. Movement quality can be changed by pain, tissue and joint changes, and learned responses. Willingness to move again reflects not only pain but also psychosocial factors. Performing a passive movement allows the client's muscles to relax, while the joint and other tissues move normally. For this reason passive movements can more accurately reflect potential injury to the joint structures than to the contracting muscles. Emphasis is placed upon these muscles by using a resisted movement. For this we choose an isometric contraction where the muscle contracts against the resistance supplied by the therapist, but the client's joint does not move appreciably. In this way there is little displacement of the joint and its surrounding tissues, but stress is placed upon the contracting muscle as it work.

For active movements of the lumbar spine, the client begins in a normal standing position with the feet either together or hip-width apart to assist their balance. Forward bending (flexion), backward bending (extension), and side bending (lateral flexion) are performed to full comfortable range. Although the same movements can be performed against resistance only lateral flexion is performed when standing. For this action, stand behind your client and hold their right hand with your left as they attempt to bend to the left. To give yourself a mechanical advantage it is best to ask the client to separate their feet further, and place one of your feet between theirs whilst at the same time placing your left hand against their shoulder to provide further resistance. The same side bending action is performed to the right, and you reverse your grip. Resisted flexion and extension movements are best carried out with your client lying on an examination couch or gym mat. For resisted flexion they perform a trunk curl action while you resist the spinal flexion by

placing the flat of your hand on their breastbone (sternum). For resisted extension the client lies on their front with their hands by their sides. From this position they attempt to lift their chest off the couch as you provide pressure between their shoulder blades (scapulae). Lateral flexion and rotation are coupled movements in the lumbar spine, meaning that they occur together. For this reason, both actions do not need separate clinical examination. However, where you decide that rotation should be examined, it is easier to do so with your client sitting on an examination couch or high stool. The sitting position fixes their pelvis so that the rotation movement is limited to the spine. Stand behind your client and place resistance on their shoulders using your hands.

Where a client has a lumbar condition, the hips and pelvis must be evaluated because movement of the three relevant areas are so closely related. Again active and resisted movements are used for all of the anatomical movements of the hip (see table 5.5). In addition, nerve stretch and conductivity can be examined using a straight leg raise test (see p. 98 and Norris, 2011) and prone knee bend. The prone knee bend (PKB) test examines the femoral nerve travelling in the anterior aspect

Table 5.5	Movements of the hip, pelvis and lumbar spine	
Hip	**Pelvis**	**Lumbar spine**
• Flexion (bending forwards) • Extension (pulling backwards) • Abduction (moving outwards) • Adduction (moving inwards) • Medial rotation (twisting inwards) • Lateral rotation (twisting outwards)	• Anterior tilt (hollow back) • Posterior tilt (round back) • Lateral tilt (one side dips down) • Shift (whole pelvis moves to side)	• Flexion (forward bend) • Extension (backward bend) • Lateral flexion (side bend) • Rotation (twist) • Side glide (lateral flexion which accompanies pelvic shift)

Table 5.6	End feel during joint examination
Movement range	**End feel**
NORMAL *(full range)* • Hard • Soft • Elastic	 • Bone on bone • Flesh (soft tissue) against flesh • Tissues on stretch
ABNORMAL *(range is limited)* • Hard • Springy • Empty	 • Complete block, often accompanied by joint grating (crepitus) on movement • Movement stops prematurely as though something is caught in joint • Movement halted prematurely by client's action alone

of the thigh in much the same way as the SLR examines the sciatic nerve.

Evaluation of the pelvis consists of two areas. Movement of the pelvis on the hip (anterior and posterior pelvic tilt) and evaluation of the pelvic joints themselves (sacroiliac joint and pubic symphysis). Evaluation of pelvic tilt is covered in chapter 3, while evaluation of the pelvic joints is covered elsewhere.

Passive movements are used to examine movement range and movement quality. They test the inert structures of the joint. These are the tissues other than muscle (which is defined by contrast as contractile), such as the ligaments, fascia, cartilage and nerves. Bear in mind also that this distinction between tissues is not precise. Although isometric contraction (resisted) tests the muscles, a relaxed muscle or tendon acts as an inert structure when placed on stretch.

Passive movements should also be used to look at end feel. This deals with the sensation that the therapist feels through their hands when the movement of the joint stops. A hard end feel indicates that bone is limiting movement; a typical example would be elbow extension. A soft end feel indicates that soft tissues are pressing against each other to limit movement; a typical example is elbow flexion. Finally, an elastic end feel occurs when tissues are stretched; a typical example would be a straight leg raise where the hamstrings limited the movement range. These three types of end feel can all be viewed as normal. Abnormal end feels include a springy

Definition

End feel is the sensation which the therapist receives from a joint when it moves as far as it can (i.e. to its end range). It can be normal (healthy) or abnormal (suggesting a clinical condition). Normal end feels are hard (bone on bone), soft (muscle squeezing muscle) and elastic (tissue stretch). Abnormal end feels are hard (early in the movement range) typical of arthritis, springy suggesting something trapped within the joint, and empty where the patient stops the movement deliberately before full range is reached, suggesting a medical pathology.

sensation where something is trapped in the joint and an empty end feel where muscles go into spasm to block the final degrees of movement and protect the joint. Examples of end feel are shown in table 5.6.

ASSESSMENT

Once you have all of the subjective and objective information in front of you, you summarise it to form an assessment of the client's problems. This may be a movement dysfunction, such as limited flexion, or a clinical impression such as altered feeling in a nerve. Importantly, this contrasts to a medical diagnosis, which has to be made by a medical practitioner or a clinical diagnosis which has to be made by a registered health professional.

Key point

A medical diagnosis is made by a medical practitioner, a clinical diagnosis by a registered therapist, and a physical assessment by an exercise professional.

PLAN

Having performed your client evaluation and formed an assessment of their condition, you must now plan a rehabilitation programme. This programme must be suitable for the client's condition and should be monitored continually and changed as their condition varies. For example, your evaluation may have revealed less movement of the spine to right lateral flexion compared to left, and muscle weakness on one side of the body compared to the other. Your assessment is of movement limitation and muscle weakness, and your plan may be of mobility exercises to increase

range of motion and strength exercises to rebuild muscle. Your plan should have clear aims and objectives both in order to guide your treatment and to give your client some understanding of the timescales involved.

Key point

Aims are what you hope to achieve, the goal of treatment (e.g. restore full knee function), while objectives are the steps you will take to achieve this, which are measurable (e.g. perform leg extension exercise for 3 sets of 10 reps). A goal is therefore the outcome of a series of completed objectives.

CHOOSING APPROPRIATE EXERCISE

Exercise must closely match the stage of tissue healing. In general, healing moves forwards continuously, but for convenience it can be divided into three phases. During these three phases the strength of the healing tissue changes. At the time of an injury tissues have been damaged so their strength rapidly reduces from the normal level. In this phase (acute) we must protect the damaged tissues from further injury, so exercise is not used; it is contraindicated. As the tissues begin to heal they are still weak and easily disrupted by movement. This represents the lag phase (see fig. 5.2). Although time has passed since the injury and the tissues have begun to heal, tissue strength has not changed at all.

The next stage of healing is called the 'sub-acute' stage, this is where the damaged tissue is being replaced by new fibrous tissue and the phase of regeneration occurs, with the fresh tissue gradually becoming stronger. As tissue strength increases, exercise can increase. It is important that the pace of increase in exercise matches the increasing tissue strength. Too much and the new tissue can break down and reinjure, too little and the new tissue will be weak.

Tissue strength continues to increase until it reaches a point where no new tissue is formed. From now on tissue strength increases slow down, and the tissue begins to change to match that which existed prior to injury. This phase is called the 'remodelling' and occurs 4–6 weeks after the injury. Fibrous tissue never exactly matches the original, and it is vital to note that true full function will return only with correct rehabilitation.

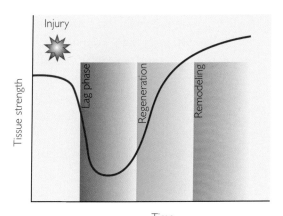

Figure 5.2 Phases of healing

Local tissue changes largely dictate the pace of exercise progression. However, in addition to these local changes, whole body changes will also have occurred. The quality and range of movement have both become impaired, and the extent of this will be greater for larger injuries (which affect a greater amount of tissue) and for long-term injuries which present a greater temporal (timing) effect. The body will try to protect the injured tissues by unloading them. This may mean an alteration in the way a body part is moved. When your back hurts on the right side you may bend to the right to protect it or to the left to offload the tissues depending on the type of injury. Equally, sciatic pain in one leg will cause you to limp in order that less bodyweight is taken through the painful side. These are both examples of changes in movement quality and we term the change a movement dysfunction.

Over time, the alteration in movement which occurs as a result of injury places greater physical stress (or 'overload') on some tissues and far less on others. The result is imbalance of the tissues with some becoming weaker and underused and others becoming painful through overuse. Using a typical sports injury example, if you sprain the outer ligaments of your ankle, twisting the leg and rolling over the inner aspect of the foot reduces stress on the injured ankle joint, but places greater stress on the inside of the knee. In time knee pain is often the result. Further up the kinetic chain, a rotation occurring in the low back can also result in asymmetry. The same process happens with the spine. Leaning to one side to offload painful tissue shortens one side of the spine and lengthens the other side leading to a side bent posture called a 'functional scoliosis'.

Additional changes occur as a result of alteration in motor control: examples are poorer coordination and balance, and reduced speed of muscle contraction/reaction to externally applied forces. Psychosocial effects such as fear of movement and depression are also a consideration following long-term injury, and these are identified during assessment as yellow flags. Exercise is an effective intervention in these processes as well.

> ### Definition
> Motor control is the organised transmission of nervous impulses from the motor cortex in the brain to the muscles, resulting in coordinated actions.

The early stages of rehabilitation mainly target local tissue changes, with whole body effects being the preserve of later stage rehab. However, putting some emphasis on the limitation of movement dysfunction in early rehab can prevent problems later. Use of crutches to support the limb and avoid limping is one example of the prevention of movement dysfunction by early intervention in sports injuries to the leg. In the spine, the use of taping or a back brace can help to support the spine, guide motion and prevent the development of movement dysfunction.

Early stage rehab (0–14 days) focuses on the basic fitness components of strength and flexibility (mobility). Later (14–28 days) speed and power training gradually become more important and movements become more functional, beginning to mimic standard tasks seen in daily activities and/or sport. Final stage rehab (28 days onwards) can be almost entirely functional depending on the type and severity of injury.

MONITORING DISCOMFORT AND PAIN

How do we match the rate of exercise increase with the changes occurring in the healing tissue in the back? The key here is feedback from injury. You must continually monitor the effect exercise is having on the injury – in short, listen to your body and keep listening. At no time should a client exercise through increasing pain. When rehabilitation begins, the body part being exercised has been injured and has not moved for some time. It is inevitable that you will feel some discomfort, but we need to spend some time looking more closely at this.

When something is painful, obviously it hurts, but how much? Rather than simply saying 'a little' or 'a lot', we can use a hospital based pain

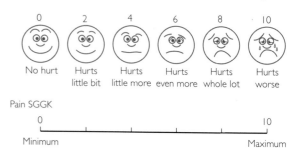

Figure 5.3 Pain scale

scale (officially called a numerical rating scale). This is a score from 0 (no pain) to 10 (maximum pain) and is shown in figure 5.3. Aim to monitor the feeling in an injured body part throughout the rehabilitation programme. Firstly, pain should not increase and secondly, the intensity of the pain should not be great. Pain intensity (i.e. how painful the injury feels) should be no higher than 5 or 6 on the pain scale. If it is higher than this, reduce the intensity of the exercise. If you are lifting weights for example, use less weight or perform fewer repetitions. As you exercise if pain is caused by stiffness and new tissue stretching out, it should reduce with activity. The client may score 6 for the first two or three repetitions and this might reduce to 4 or 5 as they get into the exercise. After a rest they perform the second set and the pain may reduce once again. This is a sign that the tissue is reacting in a positive way to the exercise and that the client can continue. However, if the pain score begins at 5 or 6 and increases to 7 or 8, they must stop immediately without finishing the set. Rest, and try again. If the pain stays at 5 or 6 and does not increase the client may continue, but cautiously. Increasing pain means that there is too much stress on the healing tissues, and they are likely to break down. The aim should be to stress the tissues to get them to change positively (adapt) by becoming stronger or more flexible. If pain is increasing the tissue is changing negatively (mal-adaption). The muscle

may be tearing, or becoming inflamed. Either way you are interfering with the healing process and risking a significant setback.

TISSUE REACTION TO EXERCISE THERAPY

Following a rehab session, the next session must begin with a reassessment of the client's symptoms. Have they got better or worse? How did they react to exercise? A simple mnemonic SIN, standing for Severity, Irritability and Nature can be helpful here. Severity can be determined by referring to the pain scale detailed above. Irritability is how quickly a condition is stirred up, generally measured as the length of time for which your client can perform a task (e.g. walking, bending or lifting) before the pain increases and how quickly the pain settles once the activity is stopped. If your client has a back injury that is painful after only two or three steps and takes two minutes to settle, it is more irritable than someone with a similar condition who can walk for 10 minutes until pain occurs, before settling within a couple of seconds. Nature of a condition reflects the stage of healing, whether acute, sub-acute, or chronic. Also important is the type of injury (whether it is from trauma or overuse), and the amount of tissue damage – large (for example, extensive bruising to tissues) or small (for example, a small muscle tear). Clinically we combine our impression of these three factors to limit treatment where SIN factors are high.

MEASURING EXERCISE INTENSITY

When prescribing a back rehabilitation programme we use both general (whole body) and specific (single body part) exercises. Whole body exercises are designed both to incorporate the back into general movements and to increase general fitness and wellbeing. General training volume for this type of activity encompasses frequency, intensity and duration. Frequency (how often an exercise is practised) may be recorded in a training diary or treatment card, while duration is simply the time the exercise is performed for. Intensity (how difficult an exercise is) is more difficult to quantify. Two methods are commonly used to measure the intensity of whole body exercise of this type: rating of perceived exertion (RPE) and the talk test.

The RPE test is a rating scale which is correlated to direct VO_2 measurement (maximal oxygen uptake measured in litres per minute). The original scale described by Gunnar Borg in 1970 scored from 6 to 20, and has been modified several times, now popularly scoring from 1 to 10. In statistical terms, this is described as a category ratio scale, so the official title is the Borg CR10 scale, and it is often used to accurately measure exertion in the clinical environment in much the same way as the pain scale shown in figure 5.3 is used in hospitals. The RPE test uses the client's own body sensations to monitor how hard they are working (see fig. 5.4). Sensations of heart rate, depth of breathing, sweating and muscle aching

0	Rest	Resting
0.3		
0.5	Extremely weak	
0.7		
1	Very weak	Little or no effort
1.5		
2	Weak	Target exercise intensity
2.5		
3	Moderate	
4		
5	Strong	
6		
7	Very strong	Hardest exercise
8		
9		
10	Extremely strong	
•	Absolute maximum	Don't work this hard

Figure 5.4 Borg CR10 scale

Key point
During early rehab, general exercise intensity should be low enough for your client to hold a conversation.

all add to our perception of how hard we are working. Generally a score within the green zone of 3–4 (12–13 on the original scale) is seen as a light workload for rehabilitation.

The talk test works on the fact that as exercise intensity increases we become more breathless until we are gasping and unable to speak. The change from easy conversation to laboured speech corresponds to around 50–60 per cent of your maximal heart rate (HRmax), and the test

Table 5.7	Fitness components ('S' factor)
Stamina	Cardiopulmonary and local muscle endurance
Suppleness	Active, passive, PNF
Strength	Concentric, eccentric, isometric
Speed	Speed (rate of movement), power (rate of doing work)
Skill	Balance and coordination
Specificity	Exercise must match required training outcome
Spirit	Psychological factors of training

has shown to be an accurate measure of exercise intensity (Persinger *et al*, 2004).

Measurement of intensity of single body part exercise is dependent on the fitness component being trained. Table 5.7 illustrates the fitness components.

Stamina, or cardiopulmonary fitness, is measured as above, with the Borg scale and talk test. Within the term 'stamina', however, we should also include muscle endurance, in which case contraction intensity and holding time become important. Strength (measured as contraction intensity) may be recorded as a maximal voluntary contraction (or MVC, essentially how far the client can stretch a particular muscle) or as a percentage of this value. A weight training exercise for strength of the spinal extensor muscles may be performed by using 10 repetitions each at 40 to 50 per cent MVC, while an abdominal hollowing movement for muscle endurance may

be performed at 10 per cent MVC and held for 20 seconds. Stretching (suppleness) can be measured as range of motion and holding time, for example performing a straight leg raise action to 90° and holding this position for 30 seconds is of greater intensity than taking the leg to 80° and holding for 10 seconds. Where dynamic stretching (stretching with movement) is used, the number of repetitions becomes more significant than the holding time. Speed of movement is generally measured in seconds (s) or milliseconds (ms), while power as a subdivision of speed includes a recording of resistance used. Skill activities are usually recorded by describing the exercise in terms of complexity and using a binary pass/fail score. Similarly, exercise specificity may be recorded as pass or fail, while psychological factors (spirit) are often recorded by interview and questionnaire.

DEFINE OUTCOME MEASURES

An outcome measure is really a standard against which rehabilitation can be measured. How do we know that the rehab programme we have given a client has been effective? We certainly need to measure something before and after the programme to track improvement and may even choose to measure during the programme. An example of an outcome measure could be the number of painkillers that a client is taking; if these reduce it would indicate that pain is lessening. It could be walking distance with a knee injury, or lifting capacity with a back injury. The key is that the outcome measure has to be relevant to the client. It is no good saying that pain has reduced and discharging the client if the client's main concern was numbness in their leg. For this reason we normally use a Patient Reported Outcome

Measure (PROM). These are usually standard hospital forms which measure changes in mobility, self-care, usual activities, pain and anxiety.

To really be specific to what is important to your client you may choose to let them define what they want measured and then get them to measure it. One of the standard hospital tests to do this is called Measure Yourself Medical Outcome Profile (or MYMOP, see Patterson 1996). This questionnaire asks your client to define two symptoms which affect them most, and one activity which is important to them. It also asks them to rate their general feeling of wellbeing during the preceding week. The MYMOP form is available as a free download from this site: http://sites.pcmd.ac.uk/mymop/files/MYMOP_questionnaire_initial_form.pdf.

You may feel that you do not need to be this specific if say you are working with a personal training client. However, it is important to measure and record outcomes so you can review your work in the future. In addition, as part of good recordkeeping the outcome you achieve should be recorded on your client's records together with full details of the contents of the rehabilitation programme.

General health outcome questionnaires can be used before and after treatment, and typical examples include the Roland and Morris disability questionnaire, which is used regularly in hospitals and research studies. This is available to download at http://www.rmdq.org.

FURTHER READING

CSP (2004) Briefing paper PA 60 (Chartered Society of Physiotherapy, London).

Gaskell, L. (2008) 'Musculoskeletal assessment'. In Porter, S. (ed.) *Tidy's Physiotherapy* (Churchill Livingstone, Edinburgh).

Higgs, J., Jones, M. A., Loftus, S. and Christensen, N. (2008) *Clinical Reasoning in the Health Professions* (3rd edition) (Elsevier, Oxford).

Jones, M. (1992) 'Clinical reasoning in manual therapy'. *Physical Therapy* 72(12): 875–884.

LeMoon, K. (2008) 'Clinical reasoning in massage therapy'. *International Journal Of Therapeutic Massage and Bodywork* 1(1): 12–18.

Paterson, C. (1996) 'Measuring outcome in primary care: a patient-generated measure, MYMOP, compared to the SF-36 health survey'. *British Medical Journal* 312: 1016–20.

CONSTRUCTING A BACK REHABILITATION PROGRAMME

6

Having assessed posture in the standing position, we now move into the clinic to perform specific tests of muscle imbalance and then to target local body parts with focused exercises. A back rehabilitation progamme can be usefully split into three stages: stage one focuses on correcting movement dysfunction and re-educating core stabilising muscles. This is covered in this chapter, and in chapters 5 and 6. Stage two sees a progression of exercise to build back fitness. The aim here is to use the core muscles to stabilise the spine against reactive forces imposed by movement of the arms and legs, and to further strengthen the trunk muscles themselves using an increased resistance, this is covered in chapter 7. Stage three focuses on functional rehabilitation, which we will cover in chapter 8.

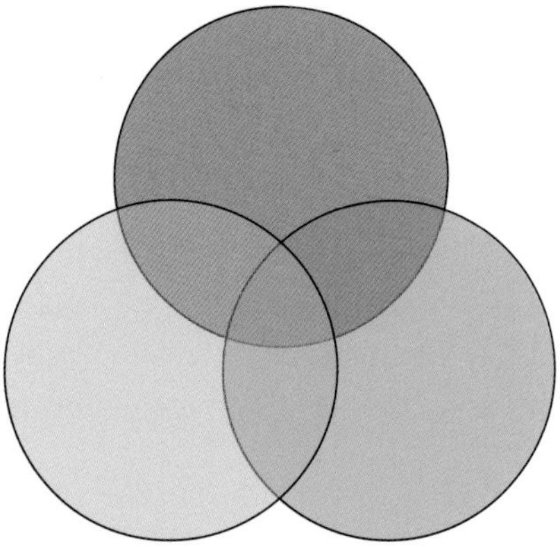

Figure 6.1 The overall structure of a back rehabilitation programme

(i) Identify and correct movement dysfunction

(iii) Restore functional actions

(ii) Build back fitness

SPECIFIC STRETCHING

We have seen in chapters 1 and 3 that the pelvis moves on the hips and in turn the spine moves on the pelvis. This interaction of lumbo-pelvic rhythm depends on a subtle balance of muscle length and function around the pelvis, so now we will address tests of hip flexibility, as muscle tightness can limit motion within the area.

The tests themselves may be used as specific stretches for any muscle which is found to be tight. Using the test position as an exercise in this way ensures that the client is already familiar with the exercise starting position, making learning far easier. Static stretching is used as an intervention for self practice, holding the stretched position for 20–30 seconds and performing 3–5 repetitions of each action. Where one-to-one management is given either in therapy or personal training, PNF (proprioceptive neuromuscular facilitation) techniques may be used, choosing CR (contract relax) techniques in the first instance. Here, the muscle to be stretched is first contracted isometrically against resistance provided by the therapist/ trainer. The contraction is held for 2–5 seconds and then as the muscle relaxes, muscle lengthening is achieved using a static stretch. CR used in this way reduces tension of the target muscle by activating autogenic inhibition. For further details of stretching techniques see Norris (2007) *The Complete Guide to Sports Injuries*, 3rd ed.

Definition

Autogenic inhibition is the reflex relaxation of a muscle which is placed under high tension. It is a protective lengthening reaction which results from negative feedback from tension registered within the muscle tendon by the golgi tendon organ (GTO) receptor.

Exercise 6.1 Hip flexion range of motion

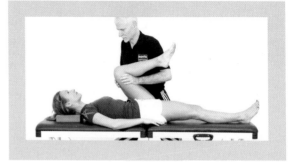

Purpose

To assess hip flexion range and motion quality.

Preparation

Begin with your client lying on a treatment couch or gym bench on their back. Support their head on a pillow or folded towel to avoid the head tipping backwards and placing stress on the neck.

Action

Grasp the knee of the leg closest to you, and press the knee inwards towards the ribcage, placing pressure on the thigh rather than forcing maximal bend at the knee joint. Ideally, it should be possible to press the knee onto the lower ribs to facilitate the full range of motion. Where motion is limited a hard end feel (as though bone is hitting bone) suggests pathology to the hip joint, while an elastic end feel (springy tissue) implies tightness of soft tissue.

Tips

Take care to support your client's leg and avoid pressing your thumbs into the delicate structures at the back of the knee. We are interested in symmetrical movement, that is an equal degree of movement of each hip, as well as total motion range.

Exercise 6.2 Thomas test

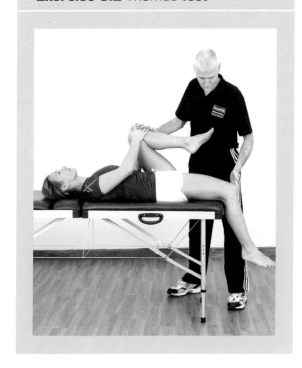

Purpose

To assess the range of hip extension available when the lumbar spine and pelvis are fixed.

Preparation

Begin with your client lying on a treatment couch or gym bench on their back. Move them down the couch, bending their knees and flattening their feet onto the couch surface (this is called 'crook lying') until their toes are at the couch end.

Action

Draw the left knee up onto the ribcage and ask your client to hold the knee in position using their hands. Support the weight of the right leg, drawing it down towards the couch. In an optimal performance, the knee should hang below the level of the hip, with the knee and hip forming a straight line. Where the knee rests above the level of the hip, the hip flexor muscles are tight, and where the knee is drawn outward from the head (hip abduction) the hip abductor muscles are tight. Of the hip abductors it is usually the tenorfascia lata (TFL) and the iliotibial band (ITB) that are affected. In addition, the knee should bend to 90°, bringing the shin into a vertical position. Tightness in the rectus femoris muscle will limit both hip and knee extension, while tightness in the iliopsoas muscle will limit extension solely at the hip. Where the knee fails to bend to 90°, the rectus femoris is more commonly tight. To differentiate between the iliopsoas and rectus femoris where the thigh is no longer horizontal, the knee can be strengthened. If the rectus femoris limits movement, straightening the knee will release tension in this muscle allowing the thigh to rest flat on the couch surface. Where the knee bends to 90° and the shin is not vertical, the hip is rotated and should be more closely examined.

Tips

Motion change at the hip can also be due to the hip joint itself. Where motion is limited or changed, a closer examination of the joint will reveal changes to the joint itself or the capsular structures surrounding it. Where joint structures are affected, physiotherapy treatment should be targeted at the joint prior to, or in association with, muscle stretching. See C. M. Norris, *Managing Sports Injuries* (London: Elsevier, 2011) for further details.

Exercise 6.3 Straight leg raise (SLR)

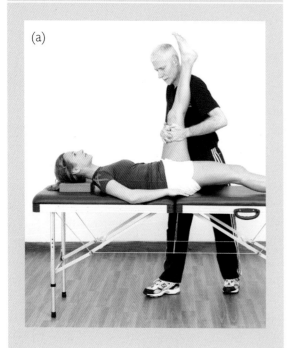

(a)

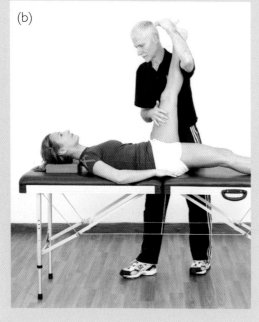

(b)

Purpose

To measure flexibility of the hamstring muscles, and assess lengthening of the sciatic nerve.

Preparation

Begin with your client lying on their back on the couch or gym bench. Stand to their left side and face them. Grip their leg by placing your cupped left hand beneath the heel and your right hand above their kneecap (patella). Make sure you do not press on the patella as this can be painful.

Action

Lift the near leg maintaining the lock of the knee with your right hand. Press the leg to its full range assessing both the onset of resistance and the feel at end of range. Determine whether pain or tissue tightness limits range of motion, and assess whether your client feels a tingling sensation in their leg (suggesting involvement of the sciatic nerve) or simply feels the muscles stretch. Compare movement range and end feel with the other leg.

Tips

This action lengthens the hamstring muscles but also places the sciatic nerve on stretch. To increase the stretch on the nerve without affecting the muscle, ask your client to flex their head to place their chin on their chest as you passively dorsiflex the ankle, drawing their toes towards their shin. The action of cervical flexion and ankle dorsiflexion places additional stretch on the sciatic nerve without affecting the hamstring muscles. Any increase in pain or altered sensation within the leg would suggest impingement of the sciatic nerve requiring closer examination by a physiotherapist.

Exercise 6.4 Prone knee bend (PKB)

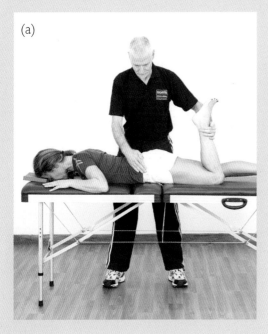

(a)

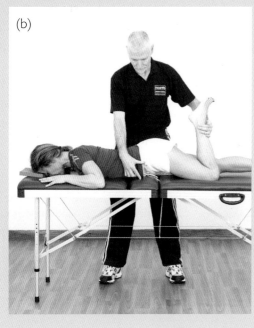

(b)

Purpose

To assess motion range in the rectus femoris muscle at the front of the thigh.

Preparation

Begin with your client lying on their front. Ask them to bend the knee of the leg furthest from you, grasp their shin in your cupped left hand, while monitoring their thigh position with your right hand.

Action

Ask your client to bend their knee to its maximum extent, following the movement with your hands. At the end of the motion range place overpressure onto the shin pressing it into further knee flexion to determine end feel. Assess whether motion range is limited by lack of movement in the knee joint (hard or bony end feel) or through stretch of the thigh muscles (elastic or muscle end feel).

Tips

This movement combines flexion of the knee with fixed extension of the hip. Where the rectus femoris is tight the hip will often lift from the couch in an attempt to compensate for the knee's tightness. Close monitoring of the hip is needed to assess this action. In addition, the flexed knee and hip position places stretch on the femoral nerve travelling down the front of the thigh. Where the client experiences altered sensation such as numbness or tingling, rather than simply feeling the muscles stretch, a neural examination is required to rule out femoral nerve root (beginning point of the femoral nerve) impingement at the lumbar spine.

Exercise 6.5 Hip abduction/adduction

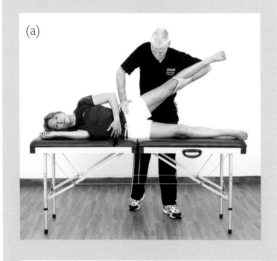

(a)

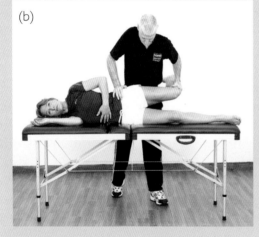

(b)

Purpose

To assess the flexibility of the hip abductor muscles (especially tensor fascia lata) and the ITB using the Ober test position.

Preparation

Begin with your client lying on their side with the test leg uppermost. Bend their lower leg for stability and grasp their upper leg using your left forearm to cradle it. Place your flat right hand over the rim of their pelvis.

Action

Begin by adducting your client's leg drawing it upwards and then backwards into extension. Press down onto the rim of their pelvis using your straight right arm. Maintain this pressure to fix their pelvic position as you draw the leg down to be slightly extended (a). The aim of the test is for the client to be able to lower their leg to their mid-line (or further in the case of an endurance athlete), while maintaining pelvic alignment.

Tips

If the pelvis is allowed to tilt laterally, the leg will appear to descend further. Pure hip adduction should be performed on a fixed pelvis: any small release in pelvic stabilisation with your left hand will cause a significant increase in leg adduction range. Tightness in the test position indicates increased tension within the tensor fascia lata (TFL) muscle attaching into the iliotibial band. Trigger points within the gluteus maximus muscle can also increase tension into the ITB. In cases where the movement range is limited, both muscles should be examined more closely. Bending the test leg (b) tightens the ITB further, drawing it across the bone prominence on the outside of the knee.

Exercise 6.6 Hip rotation

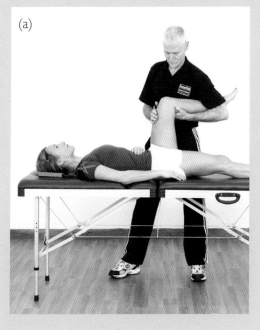

(a)

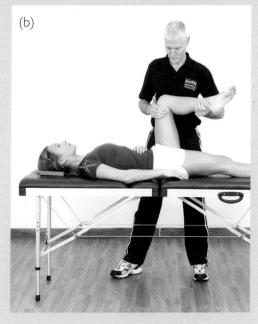

(b)

Purpose

To examine the range and symmetry of rotation at the hip joint.

Preparation

Begin with your client lying on their back. Use your left hand to grasp their left leg at the top of the calf, bending their knee and hip to 90°.

Action

Place your right hand on the outside of your client's thigh to monitor movement. Draw the shin outwards (medial rotation) and then inwards (lateral rotation). Note the resistance at end range motion (end feel) and the degree of rotation movement available.

Tips

Several structures can limit range of motion at the hip. Hip ligaments give a relatively elastic end feel, while muscle is springier. Where movement is limited by arthritic changes within the joint the end feel is hard. Often a combination of features is observed and treatment involves both manual therapy and exercise therapy hand in hand.

MOTOR CONTROL

Alteration in motor control is assessed by looking at the quality of movement. In order to move correctly the length of the muscle must be optimal and the opposing muscle group must be able to contract efficiently in order to pull the body segment into its correct position. Finally the coordination of the movement must be optimal. The tests below evaluate the quality of movement, and where this is poor the tests themselves may be repeated as exercises focusing on movement quality (how well the action is performed) rather than quantity (i.e. the number of repetitions and sets, motion range or resistance applied).

We have seen that when using the specific stretches we drew on stretching techniques applied therapeutically or at the gym. Motor control techniques can be applied individually, and we saw in chapter 4 how sensorimotor rehabilitation may be used in this context. This type of training is also emphasised in both yoga therapy and the clinical Pilates techniques covered in chapter 9 and 10.

Exercise 6.7 Sitting tripod

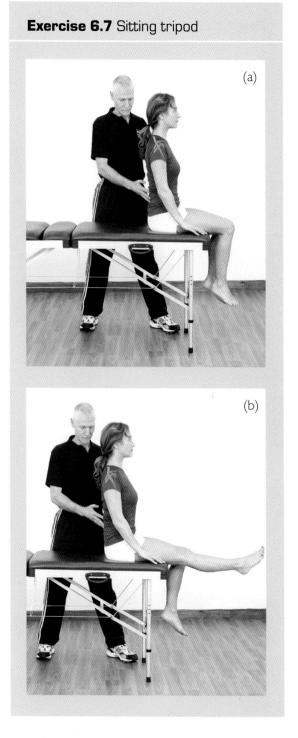

(a)

(b)

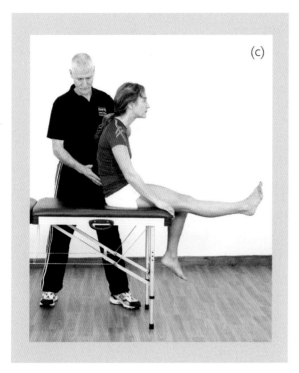
(c)

Tips

In optimal alignment the pelvis should not move at the onset of leg extension, and the lumbar lordosis should be maintained. As the leg straightens, tightness in the hamstrings will pull on the ischial tuberosity within the pelvis, initiating a posterior pelvic tilt and flattening the lumbar lordosis (c). This change in lumbo-pelvic alignment should be proportional to your client's flexibility. Take note of when lumbo-pelvic alignment is lost early on in the movement (i.e. before the pull of hamstring tightness begins), as this indicates poor muscular stabilisation and control around the pelvis.

Purpose

To determine the effect of hamstring length on lumbo-pelvic alignment.

Preparation

Begin with your client sitting on the edge of a treatment couch or high bench (a). Encourage them to sit upright with a normal lumbar lordosis (i.e. a neutral position), hands resting on their lap.

Action

Ask your client to straighten their right leg, hold the fully straightened position for 3–5 seconds and then lower. As they straighten their leg, observe this sitting posture, noting the depth of the lumbar lordosis, general alignment of the spine, and movement of the pelvis (b).

Exercise 6.8 Standing forward bend

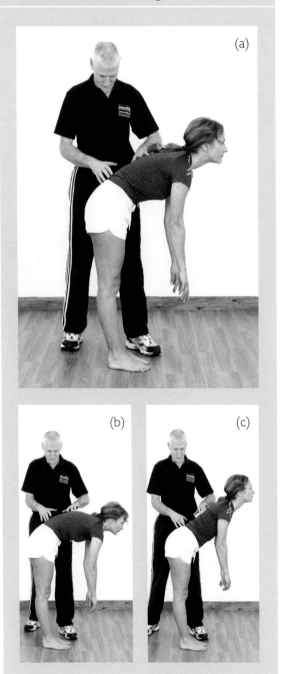

(a)

(b)   (c)

Purpose
To assess lumbo-pelvic alignment during a forward bending action.

Preparation
Ask your client to stand with their feet hip-width apart, with their legs straight and their hands by their sides.

Action
Instruct your client to bend forwards, reaching their hands towards or past the level of their knees. Note the position of your client's lumbo-pelvis, including the depth of the lumbar lordosis, and their standing posture type at rest (a).

Tips
As your client bends forward, the movement should be initiated by anterior tilt of the pelvis followed by lumbar flexion. In many cases lumbar flexion occurs even without appreciable anterior pelvic tilt (b). Where you notice a suboptimal bending action which initiates forward movement from the spine rather than the pelvis, instruct your client to try to reverse the action, keeping their spine straight and angling from the hip (c). This gives you information as to whether your client is able to perform the action but chooses not to (habitual posture), or lacks the muscle length and control to perform the correct action (fixed posture).

Exercise 6.9 Sit to stand

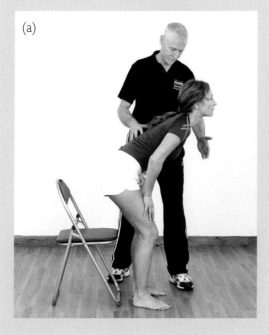

(a)

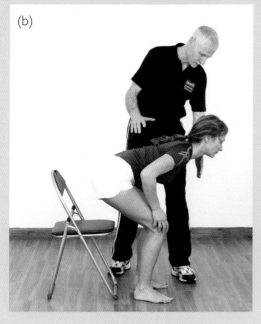

(b)

Purpose
To determine lumbo-pelvic alignment during a sit to stand action.

Preparation
Begin with your client sitting on a chair or gym bench with their arms by their sides.

Action
Ask your client to slowly stand up and sit down three times. Note the alignment of their pelvis, lumbar spine and upper body, along with that of their lower limbs throughout the action.

Tips
In an optimal posture the trunk should angle forwards, drawing the centre of gravity of the upper body over the feet. Power for the standing action comes from the legs, and the upper body remains close to a vertical line through the centre of the feet. In suboptimal alignment the trunk is often thrown forward – drawing the head in front of the feet – then pulled back to create momentum to assist the lifting action. In addition clients may also round their trunk and press their hands onto their knees to assist the lifting action where leg strength is poor (b). Note also lower limb alignment, ensuring that the knees remain hip-width apart and do not move excessively inwards (knock knee) or outwards (bowleg).

Exercise 6.10 Lifting

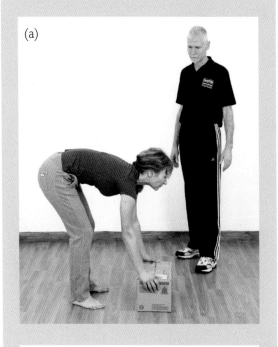

(a)

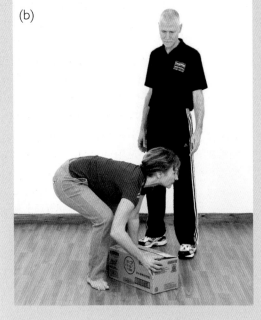

(b)

Purpose

To determine dynamic postural alignment in the lumbo-pelvic and spinal areas.

Preparation

Begin with your client standing, and place a light object (such as a cardboard box) in front of them.

Action

Ask your subject to lift the object, carry it forward three paces and place it back onto the ground. Monitor alignment of the lower limb, pelvis, spine and upper limb during this movement.

Tips

In an optimal lifting posture the knee should bend and be drawn forward over the centre of the foot. The anterior tilt of the pelvis is angling the trunk forward, and lumbar lordosis is maintained. As the trunk angle increases, flexion occurs evenly throughout the whole spine. The client should reach forwards for the object, grasp it and draw it close in towards their pelvis. Typical suboptimal lifting patterns include poor orientation of the lower limb, with knock-knee and bowlegged orientations being typical. A lack of pelvic tilt will cause early flexion of the spine, and marked flexion of the thoracic region in isolation. In addition, asymmetrical movements, including spinal shift and lateral flexion patterns, may occur, taking the bodyweight more on one leg than the other.

Exercise 6.11 Arm raise

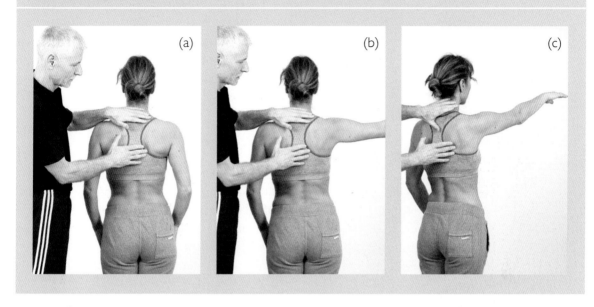

Purpose

To assess thoracic posture and scapulo-humeral rhythm, during arm motion.

Preparation

Begin with your client standing in front of you with their arms by their sides, skin contours visible.

Action

Ask your client to lift their arm as high as possible. Repeat the action, lifting forward only (flexion abduction), and then lifting sideways (pure abduction). Note movement of the scapula on the thorax, orientation of the thoracic spine and movement of the humerus on the scapula. Note the range of motion and timing of each action.

Tips

Scapulohumeral rhythm is a combination of movement of the scapula on the thoracic cage, movement of the humerus on the scapular, and changing depth of the thoracic curve (kyphosis). In optimal alignment the initial movement of the humerus should occur on a stable scapula, with no thoracic spine movement. After a 20 to 30° adduction the scapula should be seen to rotate upwards, and after 90° adduction the thoracic spine should start to flatten. Common suboptimal alignments include a downward orientation of the scapula, excessive movement of the scapular compared to movement of the humerus, and an altered ratio of scapular and humeral movement. In the initial phases of arm lifting there should be a 2 to 1 ratio of movement of the humerus compared to that of the scapular. As the arm reaches overhead, movement of the humerus reduces and movement of the scapular increases, reversing the ratio to 1 to 2.

Exercise 6.12 Four-point kneeling sit back

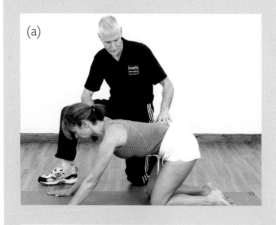

(a)

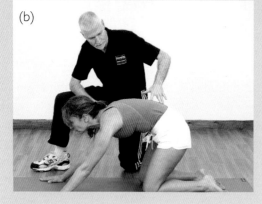

(b)

Purpose

To assess movement of the lumbar spine relative to the hip.

Preparation

Begin with your subject in the four-point kneeling (box) position (see fig. 6.2), with their hands directly below their shoulders, and their knees directly below the hips. Their spine should be orientated as though in standing with a shallow lumbar and cervical lordosis.

Action

Ask your client to draw their hips backwards moving their buttocks over their heels in an attempt to sit back onto their heel bones. Note the position of the various spinal segments throughout this movement.

Tips

In an optimal alignment initial movement of the body backwards (hip flexion) requires a minimal amount of spinal movements, reducing the depth of the lumbar lordosis and moving into lumbar followed by thoracic flexion. Common sub optimal alignment includes immediate loss of the lumbar lordosis and excessive thoracic flexion.

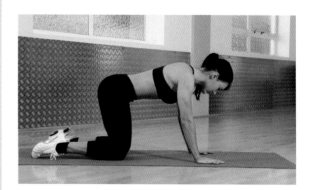

Figure 6.2 Four-point kneeling (box) position

Definition

The box position is when you are on your hands and knees, also called the four-point kneeling and quadruped. The plank position is where you are supported on your toes and hands only and your body, arms and legs are straight (also called the press-up position and prone falling).

Exercise 6.13 Active knee extension (AKE)

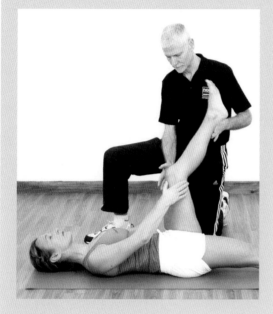

Tips

This action increases tone in the quadriceps muscles and in so doing reduces tone in the hamstrings to facilitate hamstring muscle lengthening (reciprocal inhibition). Because the gastrocnemius muscle travels above the knee, dorsiflexing the foot will place this muscle on stretch and reduce full knee extension. In addition, dorsiflexion will place a stretch on the sciatic nerve, and where this nerve is impinged or under tension, the number of nerve impulses may increase, causing irritation to the nerve. As the nerve supplies the hamstring muscles, any increase in neural output can increase muscle tone, making the muscle stiffer and thereby reducing movement range.

Purpose

To determine length of the hamstring muscles, in association with active contraction of the quadriceps muscles.

Preparation

Begin with your client lying on their back. Ask them to grasp their left thigh with both hands, drawing their knee to a position directly above their hip, with the knee bent.

Action

Maintaining the position of the upper thigh (femur) ask them to straighten their leg using their quadriceps alone. Hold the leg straight for 10–20 seconds before releasing. Repeat the action, leading with the heel and dorsiflexing the ankle.

CORE TRAINING SEQUENCES

Having examined the free motion range of the muscles attaching to the lumbo-pelvic region, and the movement quality of key actions, it is now necessary to begin enhancing the stability of this region of the body. Revisit chapter 4, reminding yourself of the methods by which the spine stabilises itself. Remember that when limbs are moved reactive forces are imposed on the spine and that as a multisegmental body part the spine relies on muscle contraction to provide its stability. The core training sequences aim to recruit the spinal stabilising muscles and build their endurance (holding time). The key feature is the client's ability to move the limbs while maintaining a neutral spine position.

Key point

Several types of foam roller are available, most made from high-density polyethylene (PE) foam. Round rollers are less stable than D-shaped rollers, which rest on one flat edge. Similarly smaller diameter (10 cm) rollers are less stable than those with a larger diameter (15 cm). The less stable the roller is, the greater the challenge to balance and the greater the effect on core stability.

Exercise 6.14 Lying sequence

(a)

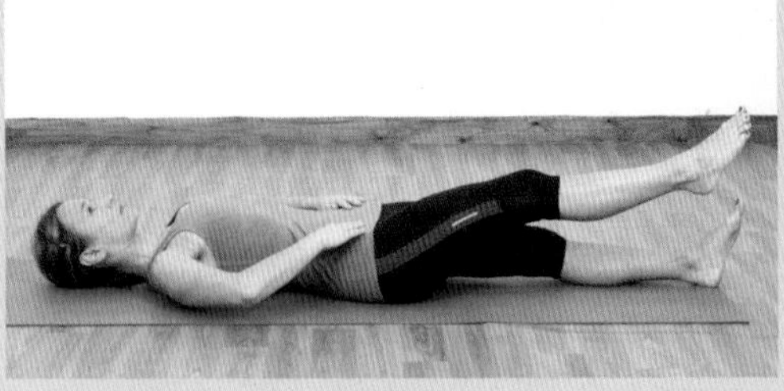

(b)

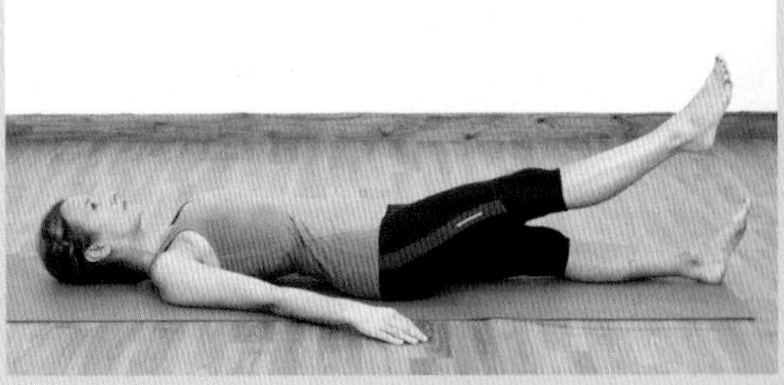

(c)

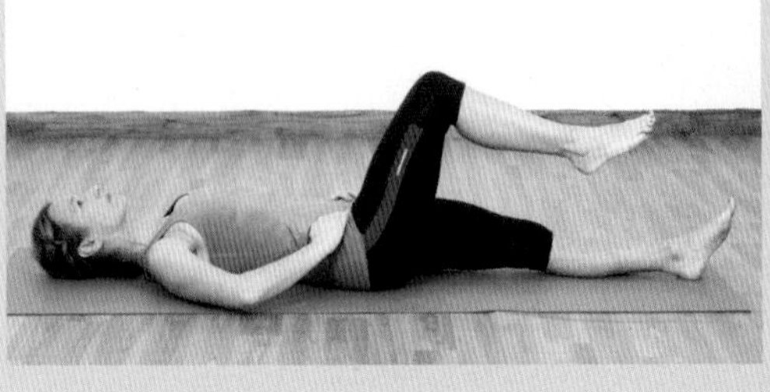

(d)

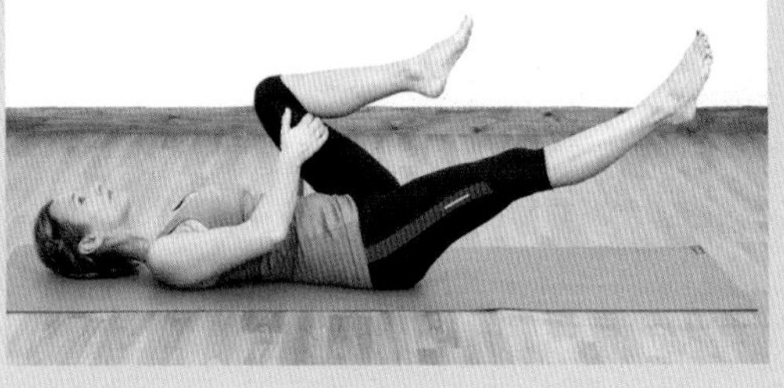

Purpose

To work the core muscles in a supported supine lying position.

Preparation

The supine lying position lengthens the hip flexor muscles when the legs are straight, and supports the whole spine, encouraging optimal alignment. For clients with very rounded shoulders and upper spine, place a folded towel or shallow yoga block beneath the head. Ask them to monitor the position of the pelvis by placing their fingers over the anterior lip of the pelvis (anterior superior iliac spine). The pelvis should remain level throughout the movement, with both fingers staying on the same horizontal line.

Action

Perform an abdominal hollowing action, gently tightening and drawing in the abdominal muscles without altering pelvic tilt or the depth of the lumbar lordosis. Initially your client may monitor contraction of the abdominal muscles using their fingers (tactile cueing), but eventually they should aim to be able to feel changes in the contraction of the deep core muscles.

Turn the whole leg inwards and outwards (medial and lateral hip rotation) to mobilise the hip while maintaining the position of the pelvis.

Lift the straight leg as one unit upwards to an angle of 45° and then lower under control. Maintain the position of the pelvis and depth of the lumbar lordosis throughout the movement. Do not allow the lumbar spine to over-arch (hyper lordosis) or press hard against the bench (lumbar flexion). Where individuals find this lumbar position difficult to control, they may use an imprint position, very gently pressing the lumbar spine onto the bench prior to moving the leg.

Bend one knee to 90° and lift the bent leg upwards until the shin is parallel with the floor, pause in this upper position and then lower under control. Lift the opposite leg only when the first leg is firmly back on the bench.

Lift the straight leg as one unit upwards to an angle of 10–15° from the bench, maintain the lifted position for 10 seconds and then lower under control. Throughout the action the pelvis should remain immobile and the depth of the lumbar lordosis should not change.

Perform between two and five single-leg lifting actions while lying on a foam roller placed along the length of the spine. Ensure that the head is supported and resting on the foam roller, and that the roll is long enough to pass below coccyx level.

Draw both knees into the chest, while holding on to the left leg with both hands placed around the thigh and beneath the crook of the knee. Straighten the right leg to an angle of 45° to the horizontal, and pause in this straightened position, then draw the knee back into the chest. Reverse the action, holding the right leg on the chest and straightening the left.

Tips

The aim of this series is to stabilise the lumbar spine while the leg is moving. Initially the core stabilising muscles are engaged, and as the leg is moved the intensity of muscle work in the deep abdominals must vary. The combination of focus on leg movement and core muscle activity increases the coordination requirements of this exercise.

Exercise 6.15 Prone lying sequence

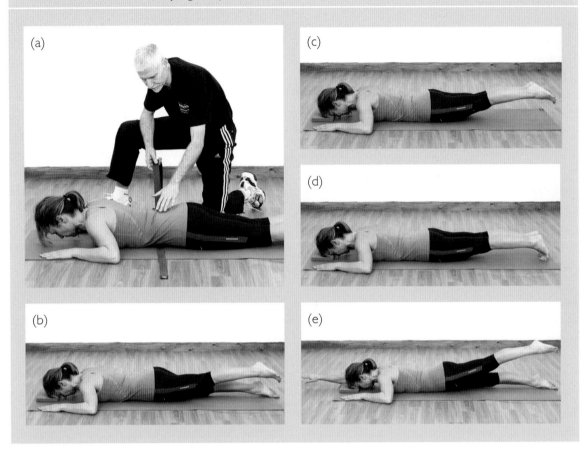

(a)

(b)

(c)

(d)

(e)

Purpose
To relearn core stability in the supported prone lying position, providing tactile cueing to the abdominal wall.

Preparation
Begin with your client lying on their front on a firm surface, with a folded towel beneath their forehead if necessary for comfort. Ask them to perform an abdominal hollowing action by drawing their lower abdomen (umbilical region) away from the supporting surface. They should use a light and continual muscle contraction only, and breathe normally throughout the movement.

Action
Place a webbing belt beneath your client's lower abdomen, between their pelvis and umbilicus. Gently draw the belt towards you to show your client that the weight of the abdomen, pressing down onto the supporting surface has fixed the belt in position. Ask them to perform the abdominal hollowing action to allow the belt to move freely, and then relax the abdomen to fix the belt once more.

Ask your client to perform abdominal hollowing, and then to straighten and then lift their straight left leg so that their toes just clear the supporting surface (single prone leg raise). Hold the extended hip position for 1–2 seconds and then lower, repeating the action with the right leg. Note the position of your client's pelvis and lumbar spine, which should remain still throughout the action.

Ask your client to lift both legs from the supporting surface, straightening the legs using quadriceps activity and extending the hips using the gluteals (double prone leg raise). The client should hold the upper position for 1–2 seconds and then lower the legs. The spine should gently extend at the high point of the leg extension, but should not hyperextend uncomfortably (rather it should hinge at a single spinal level). Following abdominal hollowing, in order to maintain the neutral lumbar position, more intense activity of the abdominals (minimal lumbar flexion) can be used to maintain optimal orientation.

Ask your client to lift both legs and a single arm, reaching the arm forwards and slightly away from the supporting surface (think of the 'dead bug' position). Alternate arms throughout the action, and allow the head to lift slightly from the supporting surface, encouraging your client to keep looking downwards rather than forwards. Ensure there is no hyperextension of the cervical or lumbar spine during the action.

Tips

The prone sequence aims to work the endurance of the spinal and hip extensor muscles in the presence of a neutral lumbar spine, which is maintained using the core muscles. The emphasis should be on low-level continuous activity rather than sudden powerful phasic actions. Where individuals hyperextend the spine caution against this and increase the work of the abdominal muscles to optimise the position. Where pain occurs at a single spinal segment, the prone sequence is not appropriate for your client at this stage.

Exercise 6.16 Kneeling sequence

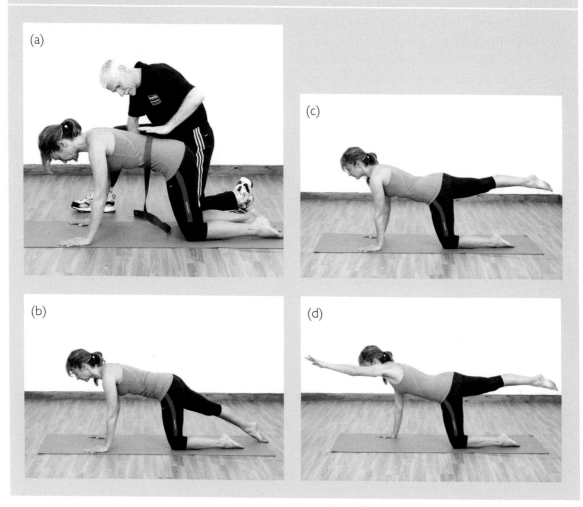

Purpose

Horizontal orientation for the spine is supported by the hips and shoulders at either end.

Preparation

Begin with your client in the standard box position with their knees directly beneath their hips, and the hands directly beneath their shoulders. Both arms should be vertical with the spine orien-tated in an optimal alignment mimicking that of standing, with a shallow lumbar and cervical lordosis. Where clients find pressure on the wrists is unacceptable they may use an open or closed fist position.

Action

Loop a webbing belt around your client's lower abdomen, tightening sufficiently to touch the skin of the abdominal wall. Ask your client to perform the abdominal hollowing action drawing the abdominal wall away from the webbing belt while maintaining a neutral position of the spine. Hold the contracted muscle position (away from the belt) for five seconds, while breathing normally.

Ask your client to maintain the vertical alignment of their arms and upper legs, while performing a humping and hollowing action. Posterior pelvic tilt is used to initiate spinal flexion (humping), and anterior pelvic tilt to initiate spinal extension (hollowing). The client should pause at the inner range position of each action for 1–2 seconds, and breathe normally throughout the whole movement.

The client should maintain the neutral position of the spine, and straighten their right leg, keeping the toes in contact with the supporting surface. The client should then return the leg to the starting position, readjust to optimise posture and repeat the action using the left leg. They can progress the movement by straightening their leg along the horizontal plane, keeping the foot in-line with the hip.

Perform the straightening action with the right leg and, keeping the toes on the floor to help maintain stability, raise the left arm to the horizontal. Lowering both arm and leg, optimise spinal alignment and repeat using alternate limbs. Progress the movement by raising both arm and leg to the horizontal position keeping the foot at hand level, with the shoulder and hip. Repeat using alternate limbs.

Tips

Maintenance of the neutral spine is also dependent on hip and shoulder flexibility when the arm and leg are raised. Where flexibility is limited raise the limb to full inner range, providing the neutral position of the spine can be maintained. Limit limb movement as soon as spinal alignment degrades. Emphasise the feeling of length for your client by applying light tactile traction to the leg and arm encouraging horizontal movement rather than a vertical movement of the limbs.

Exercise 6.17 Crook lying sequence

(a)

(b)

(c)

Purpose

To work core stability and maintain pelvic position whilst moving the leg.

Preparation

Begin with your client lying with their knees bent to 90°, with their feet flat on the ground and hip-width apart. If the head fails to reach the support-ing surface in an optimal alignment (head forward posture), place a folded towel or slim yoga block beneath their head. Ensure that the abdominal muscles are relaxed or lightly contracted at rest, but not so firmly active that the back is flattened hard on the floor. Minimal contraction should give only light contact of the lumbar spine onto the supporting surface.

Action

Perform the heel slide action by placing some-thing beneath your client's heel to allow sliding, such as a cloth on a polished floor or a piece of shiny paper on a carpeted surface. Have your client place their hands on their upper pelvis (with the heel of the hand on the anterior superior iliac spine) so that their fingers monitor the firmness of the lower abdomen. Maintaining a neutral posi-tion, ask your client to straighten one leg, sliding the heel away from the body, returning the heel to the crook lying position before straightening the alternate leg.

From the crook lying position ask your client to keep their left foot in contact the floor, but allow their right knee to lower to an angle of 45° to the horizontal, while maintaining pelvic alignment, to perform a bent knee fallout action. If necessary, monitor the position of the left ASIS to ensure that it does not rise upwards indicating a lateral shift of the pelvis. To introduce tactile cueing, place your fingers beneath your client's left pelvis and encourage them to maintain contact with your fingers throughout the right leg movement. Alternate the movement with the left leg.

From the applying position perform the shoul-der bridge action: ask your client to raise their hips so that their shoulders, hips and knees are in a single line. Pause in the upper position and then lower under control. To progress the exercise perform a single leg shoulder bridge, by placing your client's right leg closer to the centre line and straightening the left leg before releasing into the bridge position using only the power of the client's left leg. Alternate with the right leg.

Tips

Crook lying is an excellent starting position for those with low back pain as it relaxes the hip flexor muscles and allows the lumbar spine to lie flat on the supporting surface. Clients may also find drawing the knees in towards the chest gives a comfortable position as it flattens the lumbar spine. This can relieve muscle tension and pain in those with a hyper lordotic posture.

MONITORING DEPTH OF THE LORDOSIS USING PRESSURE BIOFEEDBACK

During early rehabilitation it is important to maintain the neutral position of the lumbar spine. Close monitoring is essential to learn to control the neutral position, and use of a pressure biofeedback unit is one of the most effective methods of learning this control. Pressure biofeedback consists of an air filled bladder, which is placed beneath the client's lordosis and filled with sufficient air to fill the gap between the lumbar spine and the supporting surface. Pressure within the bladder is shown on the unit dial, and normally a value of 40 mmHg is sufficient to fill the gap. As the client moves their limb, movement of the lumbar spine will change the pressure reading on the dial. Flattening of the lordosis due to posterior pelvic tilt will increase the pressure and show a higher reading, while hollowing of the lordosis due to anterior pelvic tilt will reduce the pressure, resulting in a lower reading. The aim is to perform limb movements while the client looks at the dial and adjusts the strength of their abdominal contraction to maintain a constant pressure reading.

When using an exercise such as the heel slide, the increased leverage offered by the leg demands an increase in muscle intensity to maintain the neutral position. As the client feels their lordosis changing they must increase the work of the abdominals (feedback), and with practice they can predict these changes and alter abdominal muscle work prior to limb movement (feedforwards). Failure to change the intensity of abdominal muscle work will result in an alteration in the pressure biofeedback reading. Where the client is able to continually modify their abdominal

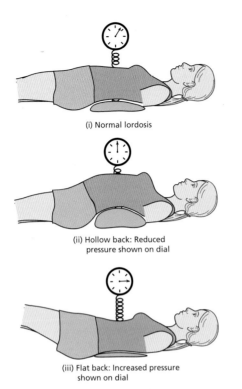

(i) Normal lordosis

(ii) Hollow back: Reduced
pressure shown on dial

(iii) Flat back: Increased pressure
shown on dial

Figure 6.3 Pressure biofeedback readings

muscle contraction to match that required by the changing leverage of the moving limb the pressure biofeedback reading will remain constant.

The pressure biofeedback unit can be used in several exercises: in lying, when placed under the lumbar lordosis; and in side-lying when placed beneath the side of the body. The unit can also be used to monitor cervical spine stability by placing it beneath the cervical lordosis.

Pressure biofeedback may also be used as an assessment tool. Placing the biofeedback bladder beneath the client's lumbar spine, you hold the dial and monitor the pressure reading as your client performs limb-loading actions. Changes in the pressure will give you information concerning your client's ability to maintain a neutral position, and this can be scored on a pass/fail basis.

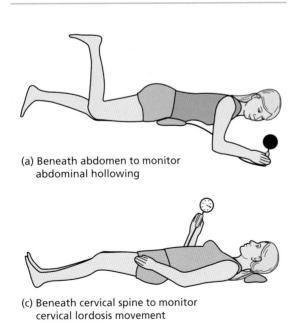

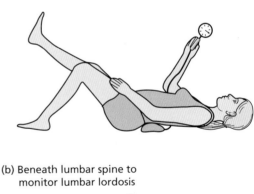

(a) Beneath abdomen to monitor
abdominal hollowing

(b) Beneath lumbar spine to
monitor lumbar lordosis

(c) Beneath cervical spine to monitor
cervical lordosis movement

(d) Beneath side trunk to
monitor side flexion

Figure 6.4 Pressure biofeedback unit positions

Exercise 6.18 Side-lying sequence

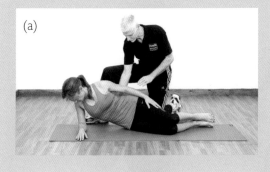

(a)

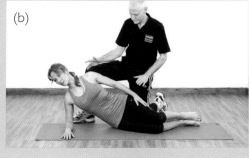

(b)

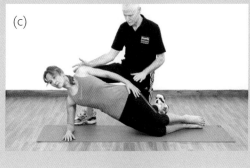

(c)

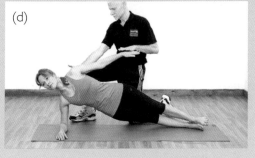

(d)

Purpose

To work the core stability muscles with an emphasis on correcting asymmetry.

Preparation

Begin with your client lying on their right side with their knees bent to 90°. Their pelvis should be aligned vertically with the two ASISs stacked on top of each other. Support their head and neck by bending their right arm at the elbow and placing their palm beneath their right ear.

Action

Begin by propping the upper body using the right forearm to side flex the client's spine. Encourage them to activate the side flexors of their right side to laterally tilt their pelvis and straighten their spine (this is called 'side plank 1').

From the side plank 1 position they should lift the pelvis so that the body forms a straight line from the knees through to the lower shoulder. The client should hold this position using the right side flexor muscles to an intense degree ('side plank 2').

Taking the right foot back and the left foot forward, the client should keep the legs straight, taking weight onto the outside edge of the foot. The client should straighten the body, contracting the right side flexor muscles intensely to form a straight line from the foot to the shoulders ('side plank 3').

Tips

In cases of asymmetry, it is common to have one side of the body which is stronger and/or tighter than the other. Rather than working both sides equally, work the weaker side more to rebalance strength and regain symmetry.

Exercise 6.19 Sitting sequence

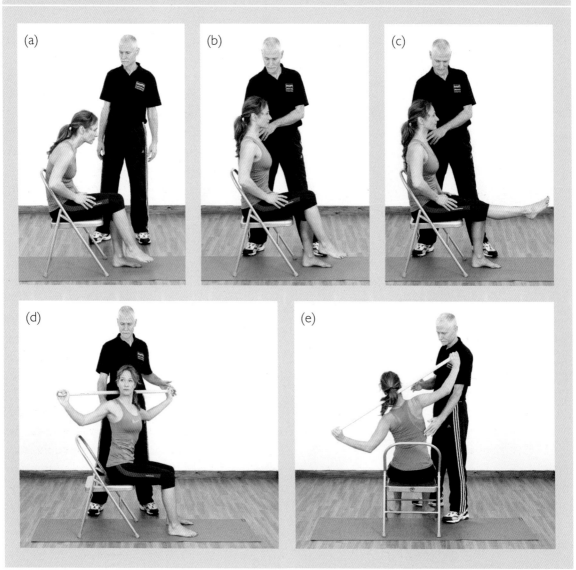

(a) (b) (c) (d) (e)

Purpose

To teach core training in a functional sitting position.

Preparation

Being with your client in a well-aligned sitting posture, encouraging them to sit tall with a normal depth lumbar lordosis. Their head should be aligned so that the ear is directly above the shoulder, avoiding a poking chin posture. Your client's feet should be hip-width apart, and flat on the floor.

Action

Encourage your client to practise abdominal hollowing, drawing their umbilicus in towards the spine and holding the tightened position for 3–5 seconds. While holding this position your client should breathe normally (some clients will feel compelled to hold their breath, but this should be discouraged) and avoid movements of the shoulders or trunk.

Have your client perform abdominal hollowing, and gently hold a mild contraction (10–15 per cent muscle intensity) while lifting one knee to bring the foot just off the ground. As the knee lifts ensure that the pelvis does not tilt and your client does not lean to one side.

With your client in a well-aligned and stable sitting position, ask them to straighten their right leg, pausing in the outstretched position for 3–5 seconds before returning to normal. Alternate the movement by straightening the left leg. Throughout the action the spine should remain aligned and the pelvis inactive. Avoid a posterior pelvic tilt and flattening of the lumbar lordosis using tactile cueing (your hands on your client's pelvis) if required.

With your client in a sitting position ask them to bend their arms and draw their elbows into their sides. Place a pole behind their back, threaded through their bent arms to hold it in place. Ask your client to rotate their spine to the right, while you increase their range of motion by drawing their left elbow forwards and the right elbow backwards to provide overpressure for the movement. Throughout the action your client's spine should remain vertical, avoiding any flexion or side flexion action. Return to the starting position and repeat the movement rotating to the left.

Ask your client to side-bend to the left, drawing their left hand downwards and allowing the pole to draw their right hand and shoulder upwards. Pause in the lower position and then return to the upright sitting position, to perform the side-bend to the right. Throughout the movement the pivot point of the body should be the breastbone (sternum) and they should perform a pure side-bend movement rather than simply leaning the trunk towards the bench. When performed in front of a gym mirror a useful visual cue is to encourage your client to draw their elbow in towards their hip, rather than down towards the bench.

Perform the sitting actions above with your client sitting on a mobile surface, such as a Swiss gym ball, wobble board or sit fit cushion placed on a firm chair or gym bench. The unbalanced nature of the mobile surface increases the demand for core stability and improves muscle reaction time in the core muscles.

Tips

Maintaining an upright and well-aligned sitting posture is particularly important for office workers. It is useful to introduce some familiar functional movements such as sitting at a desk and reaching forwards, reaching upwards or mimicking the driving position. In each case the aim is to maintain alignment while focus and concentration is taken outside the body to the task being performed by your client's hands.

Exercise 6.20 Standing sequence

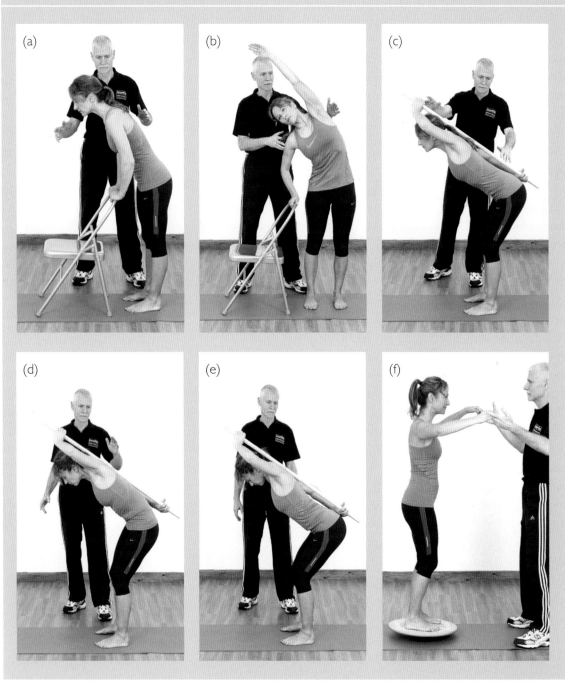

(a)

(b)

(c)

(d)

(e)

(f)

Purpose

To practise core training in an upright standing position, and thus optimise standing posture.

Preparation

Begin with your client standing in an optimal posture with their feet together, pelvis and lumbar spine neutral, hands by their sides and head correctly aligned.

Action

Stand side-on to a high table or bench and ask your client to place their right hand on the bench surface. The action is to side-bend to the right (bodyweight supported on the hand) and at the same time reach the left hand up towards the left ear and across the top of the body to point towards the right wall. Encourage a pure side bend action without unnecessary flexion or extension and use the arm-reach overhead to give control over pressure. Reverse the body, placing the left hand on the table top and reaching to the left using a side-bend action.

Place a pole along the length of the spine bending the left arm overhead to grip the top of the pole and the right arm behind the back to grip the base of the pole. The pole should be in contact with your client's sacrum, thoracic spine and the back of their head. Their feet should be hip-width apart. Ask your client to bend their knees, hips and ankles and at the same time angle their spine forwards to 45° with the vertical, while keeping the spine itself straight. The action should be a pure hip flexion movement with no spinal flexion or extension. Where spinal flexion occurs, the back rounds forcing the pole to lose contact with the base of the spine (d). Where excessive spinal extension occurs, the gap between the lumbar spine and the pole will increase substantially (e).

The client should then move on to performing the standing exercises with both feet on a mobile surface, such as a balance (wobble) board. The increased balance and coordination requirement progresses the work required by the core stabilising muscles, and reduces muscle reaction times.

Tips

Control of the standing posture requires substantial coordination of multiple body parts. To provide additional tactile cueing begin exercises with your client's back flat against a wall, or use a pole along the length of the spine to give feedback about spinal position. Performing the exercises in front of a mirror can also be helpful in the initial stages.

Exercise 6.21 Standing with wall support

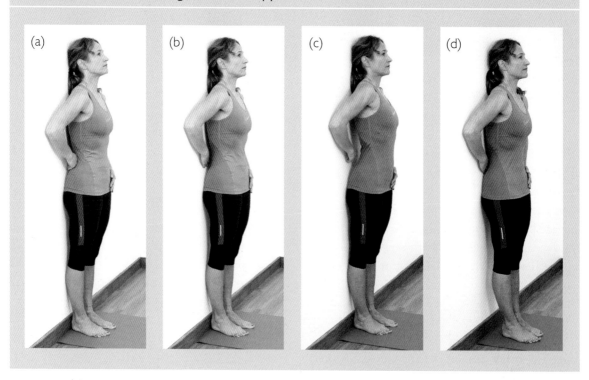

(a) (b) (c) (d)

Purpose

To use the wall for support and to monitor/maintain optimal posture.

Preparation

Begin with your client standing with their back flat against a wall, heels slightly forwards.

Action

To reduce excessive lumbar lordosis, encourage your client to contract the abdominal muscles intensely, and press the small of their back towards the wall. They should hold the flat lumbar position for 3–5 seconds and then release. Use tactile cueing to encourage combination of posterior pelvic tilt and lumbar flexion.

To teach recognition of the neutral lumbar position, place your hands behind your client's lumbar spine and against the wall. In an optimal alignment you should be able to get your flat hand between the lumbar curve and the wall. Where you are unable to get your hand into this gap the lumbar lordosis is reduced, and where you can place the whole of your fist into the gap the lordosis is increased. Encourage your client to perform anterior and posterior pelvic tilt, and stop at the position where you are able to place one flat hand into their lumbar curve. Repeat the action several times, aiming to get your client to recognise the correct range of motion to form an optimal gap between the lumbar spine and the wall.

You could also ask your client to place their hands behind their head with their elbows lightly brushing the wall, or alternatively to place their hands at the sides of their head with the elbows as close to the wall as possible. Instruct your client to side-bend, drawing one elbow towards their hip so that their sternum remains in one place. Where the elbow draws towards the hip and the sternum does not deviate from the central position, lateral flexion occurs mostly at the thoracic spine. Where the elbow is drawn towards the floor and the sternum deviates to the side, lateral flexion occurs mostly in the lumbar spine. Ensure a symmetrical range of motion in both sides of the body.

Tips
The wall supplies the support and tactile feedback of body position. As the exercise progresses encourage your client to move away from the wall so that there is a small gap between their shoulders and the surface. In this position if they lean too far backwards they will brush the wall.

HANDS-ON TECHNIQUES TO AUGMENT BACK EXERCISE PERFORMANCE

IMPROVING MUSCLE ACTIVATION
When your client finds it difficult to contract a muscle you may use facilitation techniques to help. As your client consciously tries to contract their muscle, you stimulate the skin over the muscle using a tapping action (in massage this is called 'tapotement'). After a bout of back pain there are two main reasons that a muscle does not contract. The first is inhibition (pain inhibition) where the body is trying to protect itself by deliberately not moving. The second is poor recruitment, where nervous impulses are not getting through to a muscle because it has been inactive for so long. To manage pain inhibition, you should target the cause of the pain, but for poor recruitment, you can use muscle facilitation combined with active exercise. Over time, facilitation is reduced and exercise intensity increased as the muscle recovers its contractile ability. When contraction occurs isometric actions (tense and hold) are used, build-

> ### Key point
> Inhibition is an active process where an impulse from a stimulus (usually swelling or pain) blocks the impulse trying to get through to the muscle to cause movement. Poor recruitment is a passive process where fewer impulses get through to the muscle because it has been inactive for a long period.

ing up an initial holding time of 3–5 seconds to encourage postural endurance.

OVERCOMING LUMBAR STIFFNESS
Where range of motion is limited in the lumbar spine we can use passive movements to help restore movement range. Passive movement provides overpressure when end of range is reached, in order to work through stiffness, and may be applied either by a therapist or the client themselves. Remember that movement of the lumbar spine is intimately linked to that of the pelvis, so pelvic tilt should also be targeted.

Exercise 6.22 Lumbar flexion

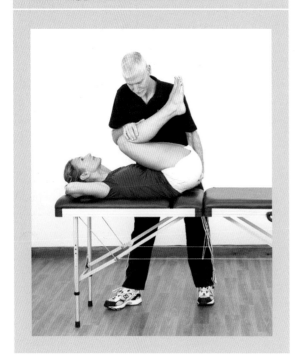

Action

Encourage the flexion action by lifting (tilting) their sacrum away from the couch and pressing their knees simultaneously in towards their chest and up towards their shoulders. Perform the action for 3–5 repetitions, applying gentle overpressure. Encourage rather than force the movement.

Tips

The action should be one of lumbar flexion, rather than pure hip flexion. Have your client visualise the action of drawing their knees in towards their chest and up towards their shoulders simultaneously.

Purpose

To restore lumbar flexion motion range and posterior pelvic tilt.

Preparation

Begin with your client lying on their back on a gym mat or treatment couch. Stand facing your client side on, and ask them to draw their knees to their chest (if they have knee pain they can grip behind the knee). Place your left hand flat beneath their sacrum and your right forearm across their knees.

Exercise 6.23 Lumbar extension

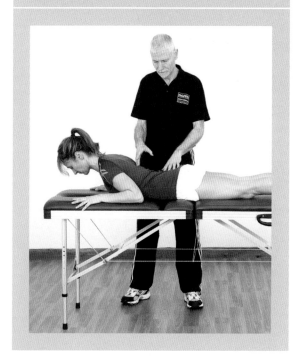

Action

Ask your client to press with their hands to lift their chest off the mat in a spinal extension movement, keeping the abdomen and hips down on the mat surface. Use pressure from your hands to isolate the movement to extension of the lumbar spine rather than allowing the pelvis to raise from the mat.

Tips

You may use the side of your hand over a particular spinous process to focus movement at one spinal level. Where the client performs this exercise at home they may do so using a partner to support the spine.

Purpose

To restore lumbar extension and posteriorly pelvic tilt motion range.

Preparation

Begin with your client lying on their front on a treatment couch or gym mat. Ask them to place their hands to the sides of their upper chest with palms flat (i.e. in a press-up position). Their feet and knees can be comfortably apart. Place your flat hands over their lower lumbar spine using the resulting pressure to support the area and hold down firmly on the mat surface.

GYM-BASED BACK REHABILITATION

7

As we know, back rehabilitation can be usefully divided into three stages (see p. 69). There is some overlap between each stage, with stages two and three both involving functional rehabilitation. During the later portion of stage two we will begin to focus on more functional rehabilitation in the gym, while stage three sees rehabilitation move from the gym to a more functional home or work environment.

As we are beginning to work in the gym, there are several health and safety factors, which we need to be aware of, and as with any form of exercise the therapist or trainer should prepare a safe exercise environment by carrying out a risk assessment prior to instruction. The concept of risk assessment is however outside the remit of this book, and readers are referred to the Register of Exercise Professionals (REPS) website www.exerciseregister.org for further information.

HEALTH AND SAFETY IN THE GYM

All exercise equipment has risks that must be minimised, and these risks fall broadly into two categories: those associated with moving machinery, and those associated with the actions themselves. A number of simple rules allow the risks to be minimised.

Client safety checklist for gym training

- Warm-up should be relevant and thorough.
- Ensure area has clear access to avoid trip and slip hazards.
- Minimise risk of trap incidents by tying back long hair, securing loose clothing and removing loose jewellery.
- Machinery should be checked prior to use to reduce mechanical hazard risk.
- Set up machinery to match user's body proportions and skill level.
- Minimise risk of foot injury and slipping by wearing serviceable footwear.
- Use correct exercise technique and keep any weights under control.
- Optimise body alignment throughout exercise performance.
- Practise good back care and lifting technique during exercise performance and preparation/recovery (e.g. putting weights onto rack).
- Train within your own limitations.
- Never train through an injury.

The warm-up performed prior to a training session must be appropriate to the exercise undertaken. A warm-up aims to increase cardiopulmonary workload, and shift blood from the body core to its periphery. In so doing, muscle tissue is warmed to make it more pliable and increase the rate of metabolic activity, making muscle function more efficiently. The warm-up will increase mental alertness and arousal level in preparation for exercise performance, but must also rehearse the technique of an exercise to be performed, to enhance motor skill performance. Simply jogging on a treadmill will increase metabolic rate and mental alertness but will not rehearse the technique of a bench-press. For this reason it is often useful to use the first set of any training activity as a movement rehearsal prior to increasing overload during subsequent sets.

Key point

A warm-up prior to a skilled action such as weight training should include movement rehearsal.

To minimise the risk of injury within the gym environment the immediate space around a user must be clear of trip hazards, and the user should be prepared in such a way as to reduce the likelihood of incidents which may trap loose clothing, jewellery or body parts in moving machinery. Machinery should be set up to suit both the body proportions of the user and their skill level. For example, adjusting a leg extension machine to suit leg length and positioning the machine's pivot point at the centre of the knee joint axis matches the machine to the user's

body proportions. Using a range limiter may be suitable for somebody with a reduced motion range through injury, or as a requirement to protect a joint where levels of performance skill are low.

Serviceable footwear should be worn in the gym environment, where sharp and heavy objects may be placed on the floor. The trend for minimalist footwear and barefoot shoes although useful for foot exercise can lead to a situation where the foot is unprotected. In addition wearing beach shoes or flip-flops is inappropriate in a gym environment, as they fail to protect the foot, give adequate ankle stability or provide useful grip. Floors should be as clear as possible and any spillages should be cleaned up immediately. Users working in pairs or groups should be particularly encouraged to keep floor space clear to avoid trip hazards. Notices such as 'if you are strong enough to lift the weight, you are strong enough to put it away' can be useful to help create an ethos of safety even in a hardcore bodybuilding gym.

Where machines are used there is sometimes a tendency to use poor technique in the belief that the machine will protect the individual. It is essential that body alignment is optimised, good back care used and awareness maintained throughout the full exercise performance, including preparation and recovery. For example, when performing a shoulder press movement with a barbell, body alignment should obviously be optimal during the press action itself, but lifting the weight from the floor and replacing it on a rack also presents risks which should be brought to the attention of the user.

Personal limitations, whether they relate to fitness level or injury should be the starting point for exercise design. Individuals should not train through an injury, but instead seek the advice of a qualified therapist or personal trainer who can design an exercise regime appropriate to the user's body needs.

RESISTANCE TRAINING
APPARATUS

Resistance may be applied to a muscle using several types of apparatus. The simplest form is elastic tubing and bands, which have the advantage of portability and simplicity. Next in terms of complexity are simple free weights, which may be fixed to a bar, or consist of separate bars and weights which may be changed. Weight training bars come in several lengths and diameters. Their general design, however, is to have an inner and outer collar on each bar end to secure a weight disc. Collars may be adjusted using spring clips or screw fittings. Where weight discs are not removable but are sealed onto the bar they may be rubberised or chromium plated for general appearance. Longer bars (barbells) are used with both hands simultaneously, while shorter bars (dumbbells) are used single-handedly. Weights may be gathered together into a weight stack and connected to a machine using cables. The machine now governs the limb direction and adds a safety feature as weights are restricted in their movement and should not fall. Simple machines provide leverage to lift a free weight, while more complex machines move the weight via a cable. The cable in turn passes over a pulley wheel, which may either be round or shaped to form a cam. The shape of the cam dictates changing leverage forces and variable resistance applied to the limb using a constant weight.

A major feature of machine exercises is that they usually allow motion in a single-plane only (they are said to be 'uniplanar'), in either frontal, sagittal or transverse. Pulleys are an exception here of course, because they allow motion in all three planes together (they are 'triplanar'). Early on in a rehab programme uniplanar machines can be very useful as they offer more controlled motion. Later on, as movements aim to be more functional, triplanar activities become necessary, using pulleys, more complex machines or free weights offering unrestricted (but also unprotected) movement.

PRACTICAL CONSIDERATIONS

Where the first set of an exercise provides movement rehearsal, 12–15 repetitions of a light weight at approximately 30 per cent of maximal voluntary contraction (MVC) may be used. Two further sets are performed using 10–12, then 8–10 repetitions with progressively increasing weight. For endurance and speed work, maximum weights of 50 per cent MVC may be chosen, but for strength and power higher weights are generally used: up to 80 per cent MVC. The aim of each movement is to work to momentary muscle fatigue (MMF) in order to recruit large diameter muscle fibres working with the size principle of motor unit recruitment. During the first set movements should be slow and controlled. If speed training is to be used, the rate of movement rather than the weight is progressively increased. Single-sided weight training exercises are described for the right side of the body. Subjects should perform exercises with both sides of the body, instructions for the left side being a mirror of those on the right.

FOUNDATIONS OF EXERCISE KNOWLEDGE

When exercising, the body changes in two important ways. The first is immediate and called the 'exercise response'. Heart and breathing rate increase, and the body warms up and begins to sweat, the muscles fill with blood and use energy and produce waste products which cause them to ache. When exercise is over, these processes gradually slow down and the body returns to normal. If the exercise is repeated, the same changes occur, but over a period of time the body becomes better at coping with the exercise. Sweating decreases, the heart and breathing rate are not as high and exercise can occur for longer periods before aching occurs. The longer term changes represent 'exercise adaptation'.

OVERLOAD

Exercise must challenge the body tissues in order to be effective, and this challenge or physical stress is called 'overload'. When the body is overloaded, tissue breaks down at a microscopic level and rebuilds itself to become stronger, a process called 'supercompensation'.

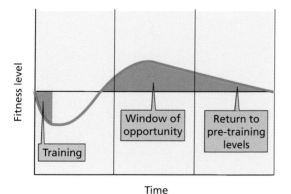

Figure 7.1 Supercompensation

The initial physical stress (exercise) is an overload that is at a higher level than is usually encountered. This stress causes body reactions, which are physiological, biomechanical and psychological in nature. Immediately after training, fatigue in all three systems causes the body to be less able to react to an imposed stress. For example, following heavy weight training, the muscles feel exhausted and the mind lacks motivation. The body gradually recovers, a process which may take one or two days or even up to a week if the imposed stress is very great (running a marathon for example). As the body adapts, pre-exercise levels are restored, but the adaptation continues (supercompensation, see fig. 7.1) and the body becomes better equipped to cope with a physical stress. During this period further exercise causes the whole cycle to be repeated but this time, because the starting point (fitness level) is higher, the compensation is greater. For this reason the period of supercompensation is often referred to as the 'window of opportunity'. Two key points emerge from this process. The first is that the body has to be given the opportunity to adapt, with adequate rest and good nutrition. The second is that the next training period must occur during the window of opportunity. Clearly if the next training period occurs too soon, the body will not have finished adapting, but if it occurs too late, the body will have returned to pre-training fitness levels.

Key point

Following training the body must be given time to recover for maximal tissue adaptation to occur.

The overload is made up of four factors described by the mnemonic FITT, standing for *frequency, intensity, time and type.*

Training Variables

Frequency is how often you practise an exercise, for example is it twice each day or 3 times each week?

Intensity is how hard an exercise is. In strength training this can be measured in comparison to the maximum weight you can lift once (one repetition, or 1RM) or the maximum voluntary contraction (MVC) of a muscle.

Time is the duration of the exercise. It also refers to the duration of a specific repetition, for example using a very slow action (known as the 'superslow technique') in weight training to emphasise muscle contraction.

Type is the category of exercise such as strength training, aerobics, stretching or plyometrics. Each of these can be subdivided: for example isometric strength training for core work.

These four factors are called training variables and altering any of them will change the overall work intensity. The total amount of work is often expressed in sets and reps (three sets of 10 reps for example), and together the description of an exercise using these variables is commonly referred to as training volume.

Definition

Training volume is the total amount of work performed during an exercise by combining the training variables frequency, intensity, time, and type.

GYM-BASED BACK REHAB EXERCISES

Exercise 7.1 Trunk curl

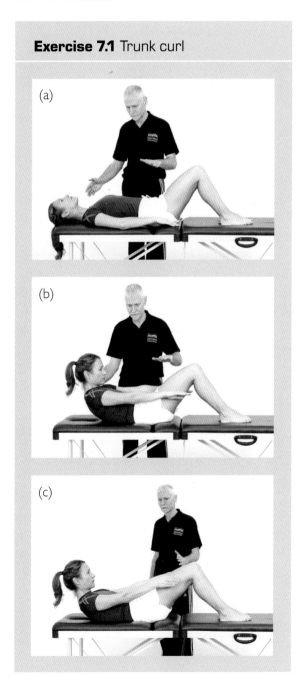

(a)

(b)

(c)

Purpose

To strengthen the abdominal muscles, with an emphasis on shortening the rectus abdominis.

Preparation

Begin with your client lying on their back with their knees bent and feet flat. Have them rest their arms, palms down on the mat at the side of their hips.

Action

The action begins with abdominal hollowing to draw the umbilicus down towards the spine. The client should posterior tilt the pelvis, bringing the pelvic rim upwards towards the centre of the body. Finally they flex the trunk, reaching the hands along the floor, aiming the finger tips towards the heels. The inner range position should be held for 2–3 seconds while breathing normally, then released.

Tips

The aim of this action is to draw the lower ribcage and pelvic rim towards each other, flattening the lumbar lordosis and shortening the rectus abdominis muscle. Ensure that the neck moves into flexion rather than using a poking chin posture (upper cervical extension). Although the action is concentric muscle activity followed by intense isometric contraction, ensure that your client does not hold their breath, but breathes normally throughout the exercise.

Exercise 7.2 Hanging leg raise

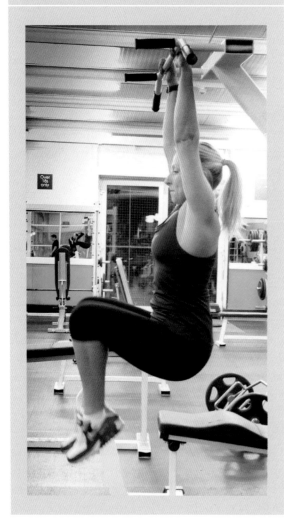

Purpose

To exercise the abdominal musculature, focusing on the lower portion, while applying traction throughout the whole spine.

Preparation

The client should grasp a high bar with arms shoulder-width apart, palms facing forwards. The feet should touch the floor, or a bench or step box can be used for support.

Action

The client should bend at the hips and knees, drawing the knees upwards and inwards towards the trunk. At the same time they should posterior tilt the pelvis and flex the spine as though drawing the knees in towards the umbilicus. Pause in the upward position and then lower the legs slowly to the starting position.

The hips and knees should be bent as above but the knees should be drawn towards the opposite armpit while the spine rotates. The chest should face forwards and the client should rotate from the spine, not by twisting the arms on the bar.

Tips

This exercise should be performed in a controlled manner, avoiding hip extension of the legs and using a swinging action to lift the legs through momentum alone. Combining hip extension with a leg swinging action imparts hyperextension stress to the lumbar spine, increasing loading on the lumbar facet joints.

Exercise 7.3 Lying leg raise

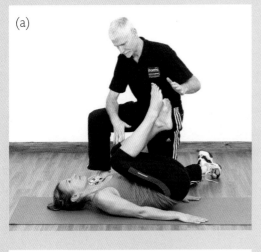

(a)

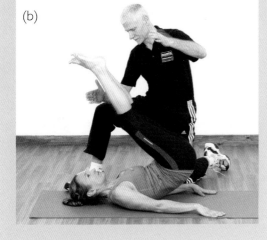

(b)

Purpose

To strengthen the abdominal musculature together with the hip flexors focusing on intense core stability.

Preparation

Begin with your client lying on the mat, with their knees bent and feet flat.

Action

The client should posteriorly tilt the pelvis, flattening the lumbar lordosis and contracting the abdominal muscles. They should simultaneously lift the legs up and in towards the body to a point where the knee moves close to the umbilicus. This position should be held and then released under control.

To reduce muscle intensity of the hip flexors, the client should bend the knees further to shorten the lever arm of the legs.

To increase hip flexor activity, the client should straighten the legs to maximise the leverage effect, and lift until the thighs (femurs) are vertical.

To reduce exercise intensity and maintain lumbar position, the client can lift one leg, keeping the other inactive with the foot flat on the floor.

Tips

This exercise combines hip flexor activity to lift the legs with abdominal muscle activity to stabilise the trunk as the legs are lifting, and then flex the trunk in the final part of the movement. In each case it is essential that the movement begins with a stable lumbar spine moving into flexion, rather than an unstable lumbar spine moving into hyperextension. Hyperextension stress imposed on the lumbar spine by lifting the straight legs in the presence of poor muscular condition of the lumbar stabilisers can be dangerously high.

Exercise 7.4 Back extension over bench

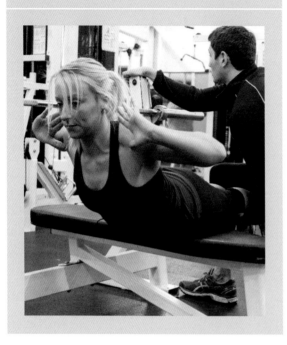

Purpose

To strengthen and build intense endurance in the spinal and hip extensor muscles.

Preparation

Begin with the client lying face down over a gym bench with the front edge of the bench positioned level with the top of the pelvis. Hold the client's heels with your hands, or take up a half-kneeling position behind them and place your forearm over their lower shins. The client's hands should be in a press-up position supporting their upper body.

Action

Begin by asking your client to perform the abdominal hollowing manoeuvre, drawing the spine into its neutral position. First, they lift one arm, stretching the fingers forwards, and hold this position while straightening the second arm. They should look down and slightly forwards throughout the action to avoid extension stress on the neck. Build endurance by asking your client to hold the position initially for 10–20 seconds (static muscle work), and then for 30–60 seconds, breathing normally throughout.

The client can build concentric and eccentric activity (dynamic muscle work) by lowering the trunk to the floor and then lifting above the horizontal position. In this action 8–10 repetitions are performed. To reduce the leverage effect on the trunk once the arms are lifted the client should place the hands behind the head (or alternatively put the backs of the hands on the forehead), rather than reaching forwards.

Tips

The first exercise builds spinal endurance using isometric muscle work, and also forms the basis for the Sorensen (Biering-Sorensen) endurance test, which assesses spinal extensor muscle endurance to exhaustion as a predictor of low back pain risk in males. See Demoulin *et al* (2006) for an appraisal of this test.

Exercise 7.5 Leg extension over bench

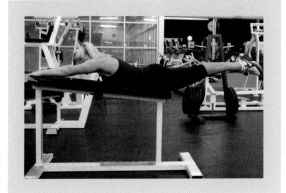

Purpose

To strengthen the hip and back extensor muscles.

Preparation

Begin with your subject lying prone on the treatment couch or gym bench with the rim of their pelvis on the couch end, legs lowered to the floor. Have them grip the couch sides with their arms at full reach.

Action

Abdominal hollow to stabilise the spine and lift both legs up to the horizontal position (level with the prone trunk). The extended position should be held for 5–10 seconds and then lowered.

To reduce work intensity, the client should lift alternate legs. They should lift the right leg and then lower it to the floor completely before lifting the left. Build the holding time (three seconds, five seconds, eight seconds) rather than the number of repetitions.

Tips

The first exercise forms the basis of a clinical test used by physiotherapists to assess back stability called the 'prone instability test'. Individual lumbar vertebrae are pressed in a postero-anterior (or PA) position to reproduce the patient's symptoms – usually pain. The legs are then raised to activate the spinal extensor muscles, and if pain reduces when the spinal mobilisation is carried out it is an indication that muscular stabilisation of the spine is poor and is a significant factor in the development of the patient's pain. The test is used to demonstrate that the patient may respond well to core training as part of their treatment programme (see Hicks *et al*, 2005).

Exercise 7.6 Back extension machine (hyperextension)

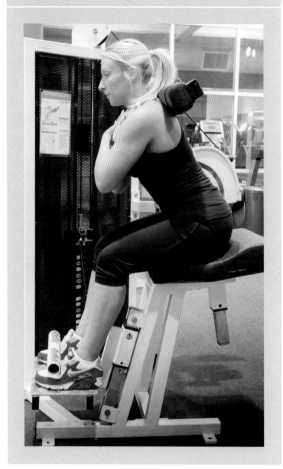

Purpose

To strengthen the spinal extensor and hip extensor muscles.

Preparation

Begin by adjusting the machine for leg length and positioning the back pad for comfort.

Action

The client should fold their arms and push back with their trunk against the machine pad to raise the weight. They should pause in the fully raised position for 1–3 seconds, then lower the weight under control.

Tips

This action is essentially one of the trunk extending on the hip through hip motion alone. The spine maintains its position throughout the action, with the spinal extensor muscles working isometrically and the hip extensor muscles working concentrically.

Exercise 7.7 Trunk rotation machine

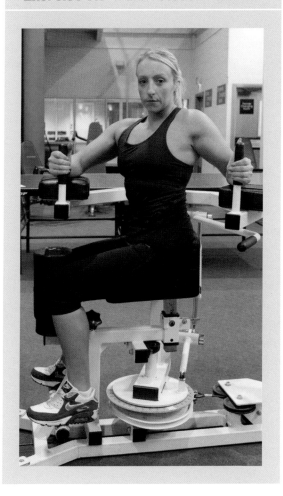

Purpose
To strengthen the spinal rotator muscles.

Preparation
Begin by adjusting the seat height to suit your client's body structure, and adjust the motion range to suit their requirements. They should begin with their trunk turned to the left, and should take up the slack in the machine cable.

Action
The client should tighten the abdominal muscles and turn the trunk to the left, pausing at the end range position and then slowly rotating to the left lowering the weight under control. Allow 6–8 repetitions before readjusting the motion range and performing the exercise turning to the right.

Tips
Throughout the movement the client should aim to keep the spine aligned, avoiding thoracic flexion to the shoulder area. Concentric activity lifts the weight, while eccentric activity lowers it. Ensure that the lowering action is slow and controlled. They must not allow the weight to drop, as this will force excessive rotation on the trunk.

Exercise 7.8 Lateral (lat) pull down

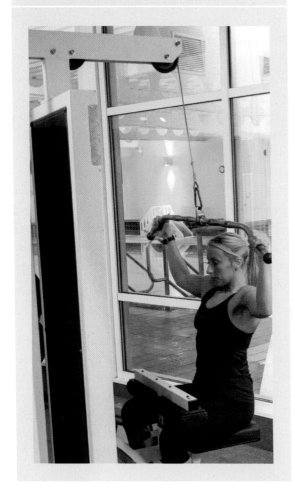

Purpose

To strengthen the latissimus dorsi muscles and lateral abdominals.

Preparation

Begin by adjusting the seat height of the machine to suit leg length and position the client far forward to avoid trapping their hair as the bar descends. Long hair should be tied back when performing this exercise.

Action

Ask the client to pull the bar downwards to position at the top of the breastbone (sternum), keeping their elbows out to the side (frontal plane) to perform a powerful adduction movement. Ask them to pause in the downward position, and then allow the bar to ascend in a controlled fashion.

Ask the client to pull the bar to the back of their body so it rests across the shoulders and upper spine. This action combines shoulder adduction with more lateral rotation of the shoulder joint than the previous exercise. Be mindful that lateral rotation can be limited in some individuals due to postural considerations or previous injury.

Using a narrower shoulder-width grip (under-grasp), instruct the client to pull the bar down to the front of the chest keeping their elbows in so they brush the sides of the ribcage. This action simulates a chinning movement and focuses muscle work on the elbow flexors and shoulder extensors.

Tips

Exercising the latissimus dorsi is important for core stabilisation, as this muscle attaches onto the thoracolumbar fascia (TLF). Tension created by the muscle will be transmitted via the TLF along the fascia layers attaching into the pelvis, buttock and leg.

Exercise 7.9 Seated row

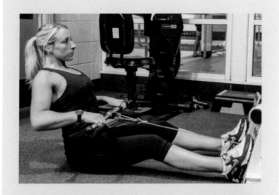

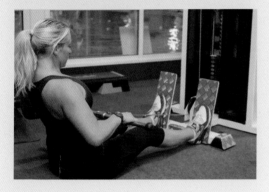

num). At the same time the client should move the thoracic spine into extension by performing the sternal lift action before lowering the bar under control.

Tips

The aim of this exercise is to enhance both upper body posture and shoulder strength. It is important that posture is optimised as the bar is pulled towards the body by lifting the sternum and retracting the scapula. It is possible to perform the exercise while maintaining a poor upper body posture of thoracic flexion and shoulder blade protraction. In this case the power for the whole exercise comes from the shoulder muscle extensors alone – this is to be avoided.

Purpose

To strengthen the shoulder extensor and retractor muscles.

Preparation

Begin with the client sitting facing the machine bar with the knees slightly bent to relax the hamstring muscles and allow the lower back to move into its neutral position. They should grip the bar with their arms at full stretch.

Action

The client should pull the bar towards them, aiming for the mid-point of the breastbone (ster-

Exercise 7.10 Dumbbell side bend

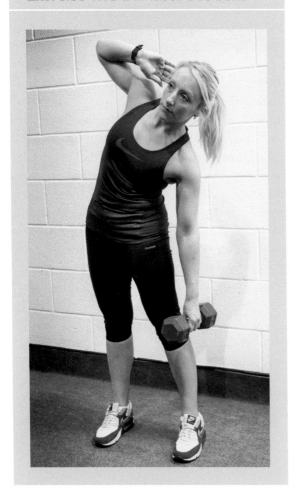

Action

The client should side-bend to the left lowering the dumbbell down the side of the left leg, pause and then side-bend to the right drawing the dumbbell upwards and aiming the right elbow towards the outside of the right knee. Instruct the client to perform 8–10 repetitions, then swap the dumbbell to the other hand and reverse the movement.

Tips

This exercise should be pure side flexion with no trunk flexion or rotation. Encourage your client to imagine they are sandwiched between two sheets of glass and are unable to move forwards or backwards, only sideways. It is common for the flexibility on one side of the body to be less than that on the other. For this reason, when lowering the dumbbell it may reach further down the leg on one side than the other. Over time this should correct itself and restore symmetry of motion range.

Purpose

To strengthen the trunk side flexor muscles and regain muscular symmetry.

Preparation

The client should stand with feet hip-width apart, holding a dumbbell in their left hand. They should place their right hand behind their head.

Exercise 7.11 Dead lift

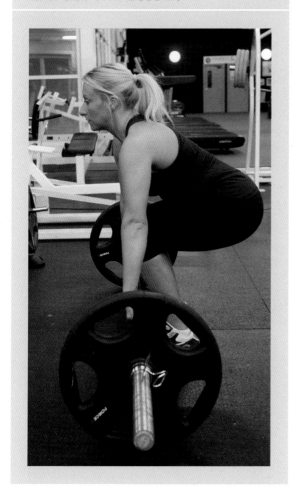

Purpose

To strengthen the hip and back extensor muscles in a functional lifting pattern.

Preparation

Begin with a barbell placed on the floor so that the bar rests on your client's lower shin, or with the barbell placed on lifts, positioned at the upper shin. Feet should be hip-width apart and knees bent. The client should grip the bar with an overgrasp, straighten their back and retract their shoulders, while looking forwards.

Action

The client should lift the bar by simultaneously straightening their legs and drawing their trunk from the forward leaning position to vertical. The bar should move vertically almost touching the thighs as it ascends. The client should pause in the upper position and lower the bar under control by bending the knees and angling the trunk forwards. Again the path of the bar is vertical, almost scraping the thighs. Lifting the bar from the floor is a full range movement.

Where a client has difficulty performing this movement without flexing the spine, ask them to perform a limited range dead lift by lifting the bar above floor level by placing each weight disc on a box or the bar itself on a gym bench. In this position the bar should begin touching the client's upper shin.

Tips

The aim of this exercise, as well as enhancing strength to the hip and spinal extensors for lifting, is to rehearse the correct lifting motion. Stress on the lumbar spine is lessened when an object is lifted keeping it close in to the body's centre of gravity (this lies level with the sacrum). A poor lifting action would be one where the legs remain straight, the trunk angles forwards and bends, and the bar is lifted at a distance from the body's centre of gravity, introducing a leverage force. A good lifting action relies on power generated from the bent legs, core stability from a neutral spine, and a reduction in leverage forces from the object by drawing it in towards the body's centre of gravity.

Exercise 7.12 Squat

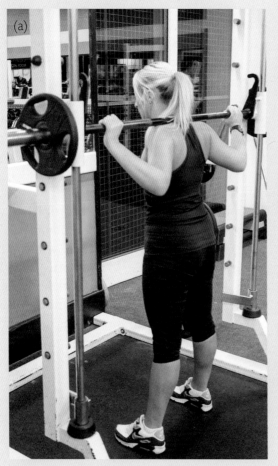

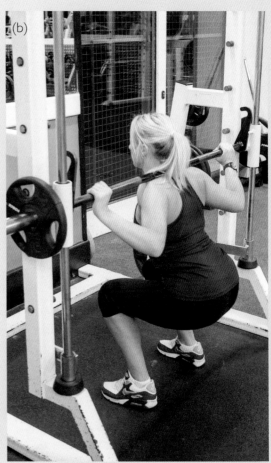

Purpose

To strengthen the legs and lower back muscles in a functional movement while maintaining optimal body alignment.

Preparation

Your client should begin standing with their feet shoulder-width apart, toes turned out slightly (10 to 15°). They should position the weight bar across their shoulders or the top of the chest using a shoulder pad if required, and hold the bar in an overgrasp on either side.

Action

With the bar across the shoulders, the client should grip it using an overgrasp about twice shoulder-width apart. Instruct your client to draw their shoulder blades backwards (retraction), lift their chest (sternal lift action), and gently draw their abdominal muscles in (abdominal hollowing). Maintaining this stable core they should bend their knees and lower their body until their thighs reach the parallel position. They should pause in this lower position and then lift back into the start position.

With the bar across the top of the chest, gripping it undergrasp with the elbows pressed forwards and forearm parallel. The client should retract their shoulder blades, lift their chest, and perform the abdominal hollow as above, while maintaining this stable core and keeping the bar rested on the shelf formed by the shoulders and upper chest. They should bend their knees and lower their body, making sure that the bar descends vertically, until their thighs reach the parallel position, and pause in this lower position before lifting back into the start position.

Tips

To maintain lower limb alignment ensure that your client's knees pass forwards and slightly outwards taking the bodyweight slightly towards the outer aspect of the feet, to avoid a 'knock knee' position. Make sure that the client keeps their chest high to avoid upper thoracic flexion and round back posture. Instruct your client to avoid leaning their weight forwards and pressing onto their toes. To ensure they are not pressing with their toes, instruct them to take their weight back onto their heels by lifting their toes slightly before they move the bar, and place them back onto the floor as the squat begins.

Where there is a marked tendency to lean forwards during the action the squat exercise is better performed using a frame (called a 'Smith frame') to guide the weight. With an inexperienced user place a chair or gym bench behind them so that they may squat down to this level touching their buttocks to the bench to provide a relaxation stop and aid confidence. To enable them to perform a full squat use a lighter weight and continue the movement until their buttocks come close to their heels.

Exercise 7.13 Lunge

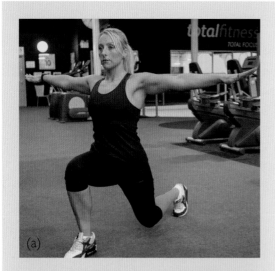

(a)

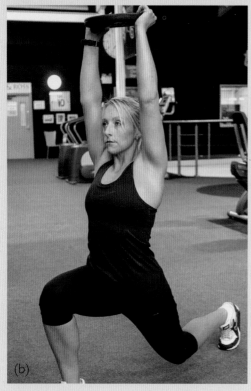

(b)

Purpose

To strengthen the leg musculature maintaining optimal lower limb alignment.

Preparation

The client should begin standing with their feet slightly wider than shoulder-width apart, and parallel. Hands should be by their sides or extended sideways into a T-shape for balance.

Action

To perform the standard lunge, the client steps forwards with their right leg, bending their right knee and lowering the left knee towards the floor, pausing just before the knee touches the floor and pressing back to the standing position. Return the right leg to the starting position and repeat the action leading with the left.

To perform the overhead lunge, the client should hold a weight disc or dumbbell in both hands overhead throughout the exercise. They should step forwards as above, bending their knee and lowering it towards the floor, making sure that their hands stay overhead and do not angle forwards. Again, they should pause just before their knee touches the floor and press back to the standing position and repeat with the other leg leading.

Tips

As the client is stepping forward ensure that their trunk remains upright, and that they bend their leading leg to 90° only so that their knee rests directly above their ankle rather than in front of it. To help keep the chest trunk upright in the standard lunge, they should place their hands behind their head throughout the movement.

Exercise 7.14 Push press

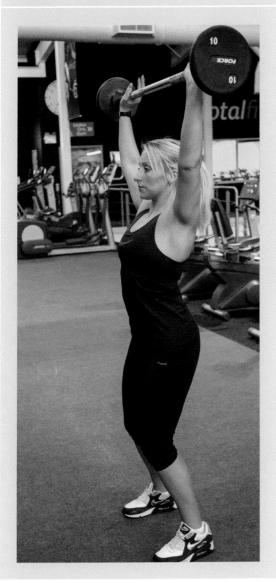

Purpose
To exercise the shoulder and arm muscles on a stable core.

Preparation
Begin with the client holding the bar with their hands one-and-a-half times shoulder-width apart, undergrasp. The bar should rest on the top of the chest (upper sternum) and the feet should be hip-width apart. The spine should be in its neutral position, with core muscles active.

Action
Pressing the bar overhead, your client should keep it close to their face in a vertical path. Instruct them to lock their arms and hold the overhead position before lowering the bar back to the starting position. When lifting a heavy weight they may begin the action by dipping the knees to cause upward movement of the bar and then lowering the bar from its top position onto soft knees to absorb shock.

Tips
As the bar is pressed overhead there is a tendency to extend the spine excessively. To counteract this, your client should activate the core muscles together with the rectus abdominis and flatten the lumbar lordosis slightly. If you see their low back hollowing get them to move one foot forward and the other back to create a wider base of support, and sink further down with their knees to take the weight and create more power from their legs.

Exercise 7.15 Clean

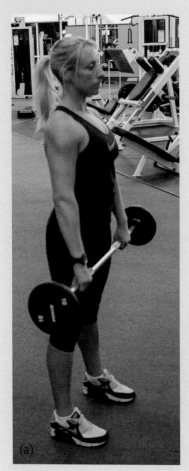

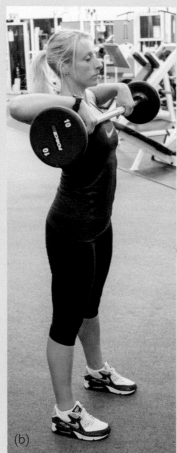

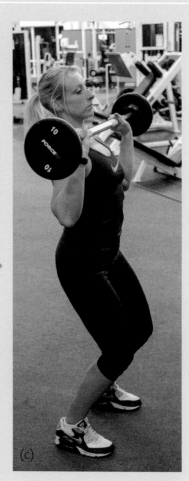

(a)

(b)

(c)

Purpose

To simultaneously produce power from the leg and trunk muscles in a single explosive action upon a stable core.

Preparation

The client begins with the feet hip-width apart and the barbell resting at mid-thigh level (hang clean) or on the floor (power clean). They should grasp the bar overgrasp with their hands slightly wider than shoulder-width apart. They can set their core stability by retracting and depressing the shoulder blades and drawing the abdominal muscles in slightly.

Action

For the hang clean action, the client should angle their body forwards to 34–45° and bend their knees. Keeping the spine straight they simultaneously extend their legs and trunk to the vertical position and plantarflex their ankles to come up onto their toes. As the bar lifts through a vertical path (phase 1: upward movement) and gets towards the top of its movement, continue its vertical path by shrugging the shoulders. At the top of the movement (phase 2: catch) the user should dip beneath the bar flexing their legs and dropping their elbows beneath the bar, forcing their wrists into extension to allow the bar to rest on the horizontal part of the palms. The elbow should now point directly forwards and the bar should be resting on the anterior aspect of the shoulders. As the bar lowers onto the shoulders, your client should slightly flex the knees and hips to absorb shock and prevent a sudden jolt as the band bar lands (phase 3: descent).

For the power clean, the barbell is positioned on the floor with the user standing behind it, feet shoulder-width apart, and the bar pulled close in towards the lower shins. The user squats down towards the bar holding it overgrasp so that the knees pass over the centre of the feet and cover the bar. In a single action the user extends the knees, moving the hips forward and raising the shoulders so that the bar stays close to its vertical alignment and the heels remain on the ground. The user should keep the shoulders back (i.e. not round them) and at the top of the movement (the scoop) thrust their hips forwards and continue the bar's motion as for the hang clean above.

Tips

The clean actions require a combination of strength, timing and skill. Initially a client should practise both the hang clean and power clean actions using a light bar with no weights attached.

Once the movement has been learnt weight can be added to provide resistance. Common errors include reducing the base of support by lifting the heels, allowing the bar to move forwards of a vertical line, rounding the upper spine and mistiming components of the action.

Exercise 7.16 Lying barbell row

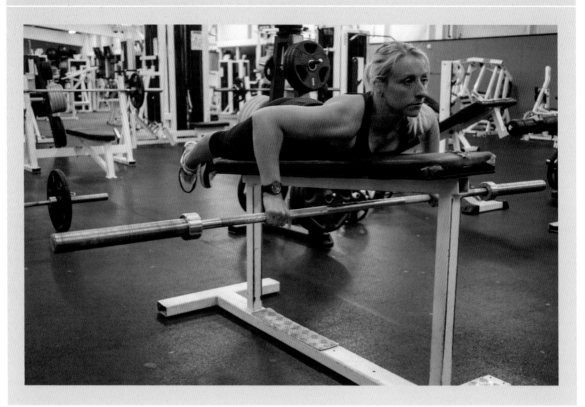

Purpose

To strengthen the shoulder extensor and retractor muscles in combination with the thoracic extensors (erector spinae).

Preparation

Begin with your client lying face down on a gym bench with a barbell positioned beneath the bench at chest level. The barbell should be gripped at about 1.5 times shoulder width.

Action

Your client should pull the barbell towards the underside of the bench to chest level, pulling the shoulder blades down (depression) and together (retraction). The inner range position is held for 3–5 seconds and then released.

Tips

If your client is very round shouldered and their thoracic spine is markedly flexed in the prone lying position, place a foam wedge or folded towel beneath their chest or breastbone level to optimise their posture.

FUNCTIONAL RETRAINING FOR THE BACK

8

We saw in chapter 6 that the back rehabilitation programme is broken up into three stages for convenience of description (see p. 95, fig. 6.1). In stage one we focused on correcting movement dysfunction and re-educating the core muscles (chapters 4–6), in stage two the exercises were progressed to build back fitness (chapter 7). Now, in stage three our aim is to focus on functional rehabilitation.

We saw in chapter 4 that functional training uses exercises which largely mimic common day-to-day activities. This type of training differs from traditional exercise, which often uses movements that exist in the gym alone. Functional movements are often whole-body actions involving several joints and muscle groups at the same time. Because of this the amount of coordination and skill required is much higher, and learning these skills is an integral part of the training: in this context, movement quality (how well an exercise is performed) is more important than movement quantity (weight, sets and reps).

Although functional training has become something of a fashion in sport recently, it actually has its roots in rehabilitation. Functional training was originally used within physiotherapy to retrain patients who had movement disorders

(for example after experiencing strokes). Rather than focusing on individual muscles the emphasis was on the patient improving their ability to perform actions related to their everyday living. For example, instead of strengthening the biceps muscles or increasing the range of motion in the elbow, the rehabilitation aim may have been to improve somebody's ability to vacuum clean their home. This approach was taken on board by the sporting world seeking to improve training for sports performance. In training terms, when we overload a muscle we expect that muscle to adapt over time. The adaptation caused will closely mimic the overload used, a process called the SAID principle: Specific Adaptation to Imposed Demand). In other words the change within the body (adaptation) will closely match or be specific to the overload placed upon the body tissues (imposed demand). Let's take the simple example of a marathon runner, and imagine that they want to improve their race time. They may think 'with each step I use my quadriceps muscles, so if I strengthen these I should improve my marathon timing'. However, simply because the quadriceps muscles are used in the action of running, the change within the muscle caused by strength training is not specific to the requirements of a marathon race, where a limiting factor is aerobic endurance. In this case there is a significant training response in that the quadriceps muscles become stronger, but that training response does not match the requirement of the athlete's sport-specific performance. In this case we could say that quadriceps strengthening is not 'functional' for a marathon runner. An important caveat here of course is that quadriceps strengthening is important to stability of the knee, so this exercise may be precisely what the athlete requires following a knee injury prior to returning to their sport, but in this example we are talking about overall performance. The key principle then, is that functional exercise matches a given requirement of an athlete at a given time.

Functional training is really one of the oldest forms of training available, and was used widely prior to the development of more specialist exercise equipment. Many field athletic events such as the javelin and discus for example have their roots in the use of weaponry, while others evolved from fighting and involved pulling, pushing, reaching and striking. Actions involving running and jumping are natural to our existence on the land and are simply extensions of fundamental gait patterns. Rather than using complex machines, we can achieve a good functional training work-

Table 8.1	Functional training exercise
• Lift	• Dumbbell & barbell
• Push and pull	• Kettlebell
• Reach	• Medicine ball/sand bag
• Squat & lunge	• Stability ball
• Moving & carrying	• Wobble or rocker board
• Twist	• Foam roller
• Strike	• Slide trainer
• Locomotion (walk/run/stairs)	• High bar/suspension frame
	• Agility ladder & hurdles
	• Rope/chain
	• Pulley
	• Resistance band
	• Weighted vest
	• Object (tyre/box)
	• Tools (hammer, shovel)
	• Trampette/vibration platform

out using items that were commonplace in our pre-computer age society and choosing whole body actions (see table 8.1 for examples).

BENDING AND LIFTING ACTIONS
PELVIC TILT

We have seen that the pelvis is balanced like a seesaw on the hip joints. It is able to tilt forwards and backwards lengthening and shortening the tissues connected to it. Forwards (anterior) tilt of the pelvis sees the front of the pelvic bones (ASIS) dropping downwards, while in backward (posterior) tilt the same bones lift upwards. Movement of the pelvis in this fashion is controlled by muscles which are attached a little like guidewires. At the front of the pelvis the abdominal muscles pull upwards, and the hip muscles pull downwards, while at the back the spinal extensor muscles pull upwards and the gluteals pull downwards. In postures where the pelvis is permanently tilted forwards or backwards the same tissues can become stretched and lax or tight and short. Prolonged anterior tilt of the pelvis causes a hollow back or lordotic posture (see chapter 3). The abdominal muscles are lengthened and the hip flexor muscles often shorten in combination with the spinal extensors. The gluteal muscles lose tone. In a posterior pelvic tilt the low back can flatten, leading to stiffness in the area and general reduction in strength of the muscles connecting to the pelvis. The low back muscles are often hypotonic and thickened, as they now function to try to limit movement of the pelvis and pain within the lower spine.

Remember also that we saw in chapter 1 that the amount of pelvic tilt and lumbar flexion varies in a set ratio during forward bending. Where anterior pelvic tilt is limited the range of lumbar flexion must increase to facilitate anterior motion of the trunk. Anterior tilt can be limited through tightness of the hamstring muscles. Tightness of the muscles may either be through physical shortening, limiting total range of motion, or increased tension (stiffness), which restricts the freedom of pelvic motion. Increased tone in the hamstrings will create a greater resistance to anterior pelvic tilt meaning that it will occur later in the range of forward bending compared to spinal flexion.

The pelvic tilting exercises used in chapters 6 and 7 are designed to increase mobility in the area, and restrengthen the local muscles. Now we will progress these exercises to begin rehearsing the pelvic tilt action for use in daily activities and as preparation for more complex functional actions. Both the range of pelvic tilting and the quality of the movement itself should be developed. In terms of movement quality an important aspect is your client's ability to recognise the degree of pelvic tilt and modify this accordingly, using proprioception.

Exercise 8.1 Pelvic tilt in sitting

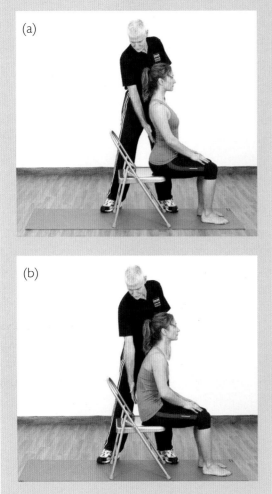

(a)

(b)

Purpose

To redevelop the ability to tilt the pelvis forwards and backwards voluntarily.

Preparation

The client begins by sitting on a gym bench or firm chair. They sit at the front edge of the chair with their back unsupported, and their knees lying lower than their hips. Instruct them to sit upright lengthening their spine by reaching the crown of their head towards the ceiling.

Action

Keeping their shoulders still, the client should tilt their pelvis forwards (anteriorly) rocking their weight from the sitting bones towards the pubic bone. The client should pause in this anterior position for 1–2 seconds and then return to normal sitting, taking their weight equally between their sitting bones and pubic bone. They should then tilt their pelvis backwards (posteriorly) taking weight from the pubic bone onto the two sitting bones. This position should be held for 1–2 seconds before a return to normal sitting.

Using your hands guide your client to tilt their pelvis forwards and backwards (tactile cueing, see chapter 4). Perform the anterior and posterior tilt three times, and then stop at a specific angle. Ask your client to repeat the movement, stopping at the same angle – this is an example of active joint repositioning.

Next, keeping their shoulders level and in one position, the client should shift their bodyweight to the left, taking more of their weight onto the left sitting bone and raising the right sitting bone up from the bench. They should maintain this pelvic shift position for 1–2 seconds before sitting back in the neutral position once more. They should then shift their bodyweight to the right, taking their weight onto the right sitting bone posture, lifting the left sitting bone off the bench before returning to normal.

Keeping the shoulders level and in one position, the client lifts their right sitting bone and shifts it backwards, placing it back onto the bench. They then lift their left sitting bone and move it back-

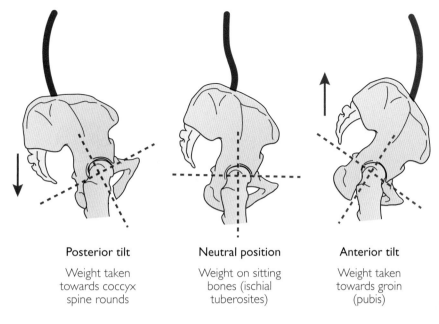

| Posterior tilt | Neutral position | Anterior tilt |
| Weight taken towards coccyx spine rounds | Weight on sitting bones (ischial tuberosites) | Weight taken towards groin (pubis) |

Figure 8.1 Pelvic tilt during sitting

wards in line with their right. They then reverse the action, lifting their right sitting bone, while shifting it forwards, prior to lifting the left sitting bone to draw it in line with the right.

Tips

In the normal (neutral) sitting position the client should be sitting equally on their two sitting bones. Instruct them to shift their bodyweight forwards/backwards and right/left, to ensure that they take weight equally over both bones.

The pelvic bones form a diamond beneath the body with the two sitting bones (ischial tuberosities) at the sides, the pubic bone at the front and the tailbone (coccyx) at the back. As your client tilts their pelvis, they rock on their ischial tuberosities. Anterior tilt takes weight onto the pubic bone but off the coccyx, posterior tilt reverses the situation taking weight off the pubic bone and onto the coccyx (see fig. 8.1).

LUMBO-PELVIC RHYTHM

We saw in chapter 1 that the pelvis and lumbar spine move together in a set sequence. In chapter 3 we saw that alteration in the depth of the lumbar lordosis and angle of pelvic tilt underlies many postural changes related to the lumbar region. In chapter 6 we looked at methods to increase or reduce the depth of the lumbar lordosis, and we have seen above how we can re-educate pelvic tilt in the sitting position. Now we come to bending actions in order to regain complexity of bending, looking at both movement of the lumbar spine on the pelvis and movement of the pelvis on the hip. As your client bends forwards the movement should involve anterior tilt of the pelvis and spinal flexion. Descent into spinal flexion is controlled by both eccentric muscle work (initially) and elastic recoil (at end of range). The spinal extensors control spinal flexion, while the hip extensors control anterior pelvic tilt. At full inner range the muscles relax, and the initial return to the standing position begins by recoil of the stretched soft tissues. This initial energy is dependent on the elastic properties of the tissues, which are reduced in people with chronic low back pain and those who are inactive. Once movement has been initiated by elastic recoil further trunk raising is carried out by concentric activity of the spinal extensors and hip extensors to reverse the action of the spine and pelvis. This reduced need for muscle contractile activity can be seen on an EMG (electromyography) machine and is termed myoelectrical silence. It is termed the flexion relaxation phenomenon (FRP) or flexion relaxation response. The FRP changes during fatigue of the erector spine, occurring earlier in flexion and later in extension suggesting an increased reliance on inert force creation by the lumbar tissues (Descarreaux *et al*, 2008). In addition, the FRP changes in individuals with chronic low back pain (Colloca and Hinrichs, 2005) where muscle spasm may interfere with load sharing between contractile (muscle work) and inert (elastic recoil) force production.

Definition

The flexion relaxation phenomenon (FRP) is a lack of activity in the spinal extensor muscles at full flexion from standing. Elastic recoil of the posteriorly placed spinal tissues provides resistance to further flexion, and initiation of extension.

Exercise 8.2 Hip hinge

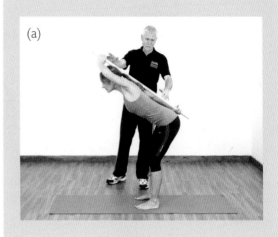
(a)

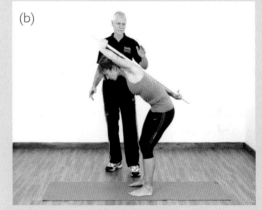
(b)

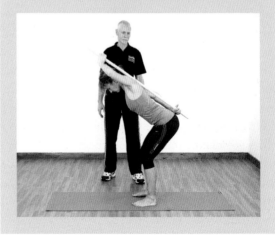

Purpose

To develop an optimal lumbo-pelvic rhythm during forward bending.

Preparation

Begin by revisiting the core training sequences in chapter 6, and asking your client to perform standing actions. Ask your client to place a pole along the length of their spine and perform the forward bend action described on p. 104 as a precursor to the exercises below.

Action

Your client should stand with their feet hip-width apart and perform the standard hip hinge action using a pole placed along the length of the spine. They should bend their left arm overhead to grip the top of the pole and their right arm behind their back to grip the base of the pole. Instruct them to bend forwards to an angle of 45°, remembering to hinge from the hip joints and bend their knees and ankles keeping the pole pressed firmly across the whole length of the spine. Perform the action for five repetitions to feel the rhythm of the movement.

The client should then place their hands behind their back with the backs of their hands placed flat against the tailbone (sacrum). They should slightly bend their knees and ankles and hinge forwards from the hips keeping their spine straight. Next, they draw their arms back slightly and squeeze their shoulder blades together to give the feeling of opening their chest and avoiding thoracic flexion.

Your client should then place their hands on their hips and bend forwards, initiating the movement with anterior pelvic tilt. As the spine reaches a 30° angle with the vertical, they should flex their spine, bending evenly throughout its whole length as they approach the horizontal position. They should then return to the standing position by initiating movement with posterior pelvic tilt followed by spinal extension in a controlled movement.

Place a dining chair or gym bench 0.5 to 1 m in front of your client, and ask them to stand with their feet hip-width apart and their hands by their sides. Bend forwards, initiating the movement with anterior pelvic tilt followed by spinal flexion. At the same time they should reach forwards to touch the bench. A return to standing should be initiated with posterior pelvic tilt followed by spinal extension drawing the arms back towards the side of the body.

Your client should then stand with their feet hip-width apart and their hands by their sides, then bend forwards, taking care to move their pelvis and spine together so the spine maintains an optimal orientation rather than hyperflexing in the thoracic area. Instruct your client to reach forwards and downwards so that their hands are close to the floor, then return to the standing position maintaining good spinal alignment to draw their hands back to the sides of the body.

Tips

Your client must perform these actions slowly, maintaining control of the pelvis and spine at all times. When using the pole to monitor movement, if spinal flexion occurs the back will round forcing the pole to leave contact with the base of the spine. Where excessive spinal extension occurs the gap between the lumbar spine and the pole will increase substantially.

THE LIFTING ACTION

When we lift an object there are several mechanical (physics) forces at work. Forward movement of the body is counteracted by power from the hip extensor muscles and elastic recoil of the spinal tissues. The weight to be lifted comprises both the object and the weight of the upper body, which both act as a fulcrum on the hip joint. Ways of varying this mechanical layout include bending the legs to supply some of the lifting force from the leg musculature, drawing the object closer into the pelvis to reduce the effect of leverage and changing the angle of trunk flexion to alter the stretch/recoil of the elastic tissues within the spine.

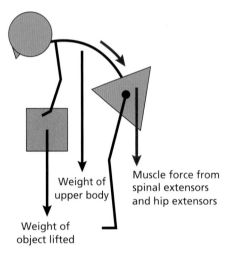

Figure 8.2 The physics of lifting

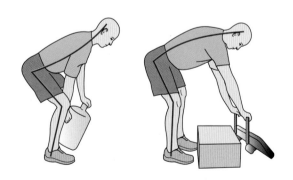

Squat lift: Hips lower and spine more vertical

Stoop lift: Hips higher and spine more horizontal

Figure 8.3 Squat and stoop lift

In order to lift an object from the floor, we obviously have to reach our hand downwards towards floor level. Reaching the hand downwards can be achieved through two distinct movement strategies: squatting and stooping. In a squat action, the spine is kept relatively upright with the lumbar spine in its neutral position. The knees and hips flex to lower the body. In a stoop action, the knees remain relatively inactive and the spine flexes throughout its full length to position the hands closer to the floor. In reality many lifting techniques combine both the stoop and squat actions, but a brief analysis of these two movements separately is helpful.

During a squat lift the feet are apart and the object being lifted can be drawn closer into the pelvis, in line with the body's centre of gravity. This effectively reduces the lever arm formed by the object, so in relative terms makes the object 'lighter' (actual weight multiplied by leverage effect). Power for the lift comes from the strong gluteal and quadriceps muscles, which lift both the weight of the upper body and the object being lifted. The energy expenditure of a squat lift is higher than that of a stoop lift simply because the legs are lifting both weights. Because the object being lifted remains relatively close to the body, its weight applies fairly direct compression onto the spine. As the weight moves forward the compression effect is reduced and a bending (torsion) effect is introduced. The torsion effect increases

Image labels within Figure 8.2:
Weight of upper body
Muscle force from spinal extensors and hip extensors
Weight of object lifted

the tendency of the spine to flex, initially reducing the lumbar lordosis and eventually flattening it completely. In extreme cases the spine can flex into a range similar to that of a stoop lift.

With a stoop lift, the knees remain inactive, with the client locking their knees. Power for the lift comes from the hip extensor and spinal extensor muscles. Initially the elastic recoil of both the tissues counterbalances the effect of the object being lifted and may even initiate body extension from the fully flexed position. As the weight is lifted the gluteal and spinal extensor muscles become active, hoisting the body upwards against gravity. Because the spine is flexed throughout the action, the anterior aspect of the spinal discs is compressed while the posteriorly aspect is lengthened. We saw in chapter 1 that pressure changes within the disc with spinal movement, and these changes can be extreme. With a stoop action there is a 50 per cent increase in pressure of the lumbar (measured at L3) compared to normal standing, and the full range of stoop increases pressure by 120 per cent compared to standing. Although these disc pressures are high they are partially attenuated by muscular stability mechanisms acting on the spine, which help turn the trunk into a more solid cylinder (see chapter 4). Bear in mind that these mechanisms are only optimal in a client who does not have movement dysfunction and possesses the ability to recruit the muscles at the right time during the lifting action.

Describing the lifting action from an academic perspective is clearly useful, but the functional application of these techniques within an occupational environment and day-to-day activities is the key to prevention of back injury. We need to look at a structured approach to teach our clients a correct manual handling technique.

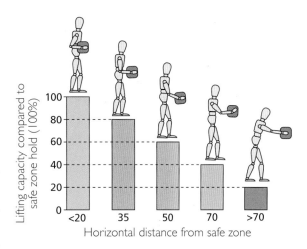

Figure 8.4 Proportional lifting capacity depending on reaching distance

One of the aims of an optimal lifting technique is to draw the object close to the body's centre of gravity and keep it there for the majority of the lift. Moving the object away from the body's centre of gravity increases the leverage effects imposed upon the spine. The area just in front of the client's pelvis is therefore termed the 'safe zone'. Figure 8.4 looks at lifting capacity and compares the proportional effect of lifting a 25 kg box held close into the pelvis, and shows how load increases with distance from the body due to leverage effects. Moving the object away from the body by one forearm length reduces lifting capacity from 25 to 15 kg. Moving the object downwards and forwards so that it is placed on the floor in front of the toes reduces the lifting capacity from 25 to 5 kg, while lifting it above shoulder height again reduces lifting capacity to 5 kg. Clearly, holding an object away from the body greatly reduces an individual's safe lifting capacity. Figure 8.5 illustrates this fact, comparing the lifting capacity holding an object within the safe zone at pelvic height, to that of different reaching distances and heights. Lifting an object at a reaching distance greater than 70 cm from the vertical bodyline reduces the safe lifting capacity to just 20 per cent of that achieved when the object is lifted from the safe zone.

Before a lift is performed it is important to form a plan and assess the risks involved. Assessment should be of the environment, the object and the individual who will perform the lift. Factors within the environment include the floor surface, determining whether it is even, slippery, or has an unclear path of access. Assessment of the object must include the size, shape, weight, grip and weight distribution. Finally, the individual themselves should form part of the assessment, a factor which is often forgotten. The individual's capacity to lift due to their health, strength and skill should all be taken into consideration.

The first action when performing a lift is to align the body correctly so that the object can be moved into the safe zone quickly. This means positioning the feet. When we lift, our knees will bend, so it is important when lifting a large object to stand at the corner of the object so that the forward knee motion involved with flexion can occur unhindered. Stand at the corner of the object and keep at least one foot flat. Lifting onto the toes raises the body's centre of gravity and reduces the base of support, compromising balance and stability. In addition grip onto the floor is obviously reduced. It is always better to keep both feet flat, but in cases where knee motion is limited this may not be possible. In this case the foot of the leg with limited motion should be placed forwards so that it moves less.

Ensure that the pelvis (safe zone) is close to the object so that it is almost touching. Grip the object securely, preferably with your fingers beneath the object, but where this is not possible use the flat of the hand on the side of the object. In occupational situations safety gloves may be

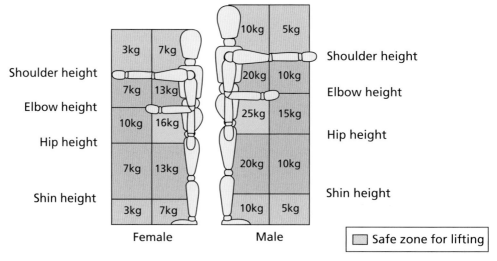

Figure 8.5 Lifting capacity at different body positions

Table 8.2	Assessment factors prior to manual lifting	
Environment	**Object**	**Individual**
• Floor surface: is the floor slippery or uneven in places. Can an adequate grip be maintained throughout the lift? • Pathway/access: are there any doors to go through, or objects which may hinder access? • Final position: where will the lifter put the object? Is this area clear and secure?	• Size: large/small. • Weight: assessed in relation to lifting capacity. • Surface: slippery/sharp/uneven. • Weight distribution: rigid/fluid.	• Previous relevant injuries (e.g. knee or low back)? • Medical conditions (e.g. hypertension). • Leg power. • Core stability. • Skill level/experience with object type.

required, and in all circumstances it is important to ensure maximum hand contact and not try to lift with the fingers alone. Lifting with the fingers by themselves creates a weak link in the body chain as they have little power. Draw the object in towards the safe zone by sliding it along the floor rather than lifting. Once the object is within the safe zone the powerful lift comes from the legs themselves rather than the arms. Drive the hips upwards, holding the object close into the body so that its weight acts through the safe zone rather than creating a leverage force by sliding forward of the bodyline. In an ideal lifting situation this powerful action is a squat lift, but where the object moves forward, power from the legs is lost and the technique becomes a stoop lift, relying on the back musculature to hoist the object upwards through the long lever of the spine itself.

Once the object has been lifted you may need to turn to face another direction prior to carrying it. The turn should be carried out by moving the feet rather than twisting the spine. Spinal injury is more common when flexion and rotation actions are combined than with single plane movements. While carrying the object keep it held tightly within the safe zone, and reverse the procedure to place the object back onto the floor. Keep the object close into the safe zone, then bend the knees and keep your feet flat to maintain body stability while the object is lowered to the floor in a controlled manner. Most of your clients will have performed a squat exercise in the gym and it is now a question of converting this action into a more functional squat lift using a box rather than barbell.

Exercise 8.3 Squat lift

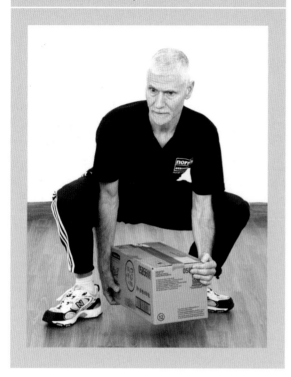

at least one hand beneath it and slide the object towards their pelvis keeping it resting on the floor. The object is pulled close in to the body when the client stands up. Instruct your client to turn 90° by moving their feet rather than their spine and walk forwards by four or five paces. They should reverse the action to place the object back onto the floor.

Tips

Correct timing is important with all manual handling actions. With the squat lift a common error is to lift the hips and allow the object to slide forwards and downwards, failing to keep up with the vertical action of the hips. This changes the pure squat action into a stoop lift where the object pulls the lifter forwards and downwards. This error can be avoided by keeping the object touching the pelvis throughout the lifting action.

Purpose

To convert the squat action into a more functional lifting technique.

Preparation

Standing in front of the box resting on the floor.

Action

The client should step to the side so that they face the corner of the object, with one foot facing along the leading edge and the other foot facing along the trailing edge. They should keep their feet flat and bend their knees to squat downwards into a position low enough that the safe zone is horizontally level with the centre of the object you are lifting. They should grip the object with

Exercise 8.4 Stoop lift

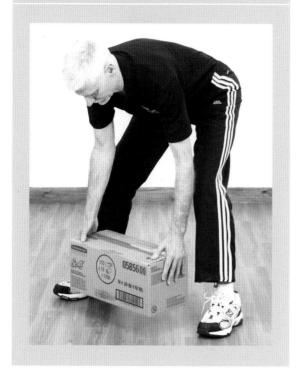

lift by reversing the action, using posterior pelvic tilt followed by spinal extension throughout the length of the spine.

Tips

Note from figure 8.5 that the lifting capacity from floor level at arm's length is significantly less than that from the safe zone. The stoop lift should only be used with light weights, and performed in a controlled action. See also the Pilates exercise standing rolldown in chapter 10 to practise the coordination of this action without lifting the weight of a box.

Purpose

To combine pelvic tilt and spinal flexion in a coordinated forward bend action.

Preparation

Your client should begin standing with feet hip-width apart, hands by their sides. Have a light box positioned on the floor in front of their feet.

Action

Instruct the client to bend forwards, initiating the motion with a slight knee flexion (knee softening) combined with anterior pelvic tilt. At the same time, they should flex the spine, moving throughout the whole spinal length to reach their hands down to the object. They should grip the box and

Exercise 8.5 Singlehanded lift

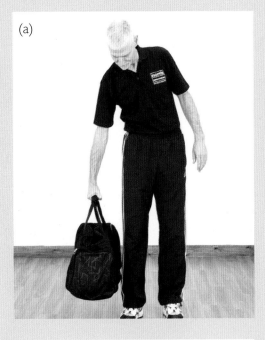

(a)

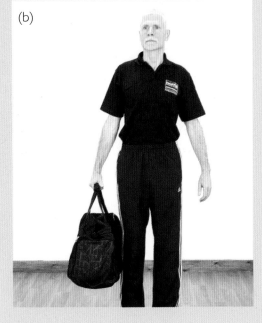

(b)

Purpose

To learn the technique of lifting a light object from the floor singlehanded.

Preparation

The client begins by standing with their feet shoulder-width apart, with an object 50 cm to 1 m in front of them to their right side.

Action

Tell your client to step forwards with their left leg bending their right knee, and place their left hand onto their left thigh. They should keep their spine upright and reach downwards with their right hand to grip the object, then press on their left leg to draw their body back to the standing position bringing the right foot in line with the left.

Tips

A singlehanded lift is really a modification of a simple lunge exercise often practised in the gym. To gain leg strength and coordination for this lift your client should practise the lunge initially with their hands behind their head, to keep their chest open and trunk upright. Next, get them to practise with their hands on their hips. Finally, they should practice the action of the singlehanded lift using one hand on the lifting-side thigh to help provide power, while the other hand reaches towards the floor. Make sure that your client focuses on good lower limb alignment, bringing the knee over the foot rather than allowing it to sway inward or outward.

Exercise 8.6 Stage lift

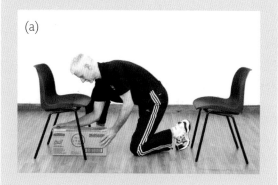

(a)

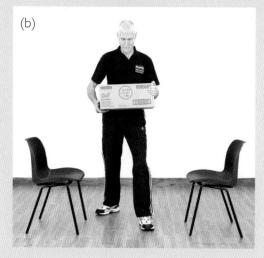

(b)

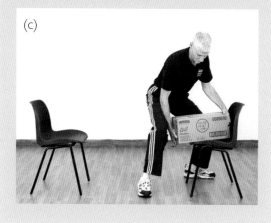

(c)

Purpose
To combine several individual movements into a smooth manual handling technique.

Preparation
Begin with a small object placed beneath the gym bench, and a second gym bench placed 3 to 5 m away.

Action
For the first action have your client kneel down and pull the object from underneath the bench making sure that its weight is taken through the floor. They should reposition for the second action to perform a squat lift, gripping and lifting the object, pulling it into the safe zone. For the third action they should walk their feet around to turn their body to face the second bench. Finally, have them carry the object towards the second bench, placing the object onto the bench using a squat lift to lower in a controlled fashion.

Tips
The stage lift is really an exercise in coordination and timing. Each of the lifting actions has been practised previously, but it is necessary to put the actions together into a smooth sequence. The lift breaks down if one of the actions is performed poorly and acts as the weak link in the chain.

Exercise 8.7 Two-person lift

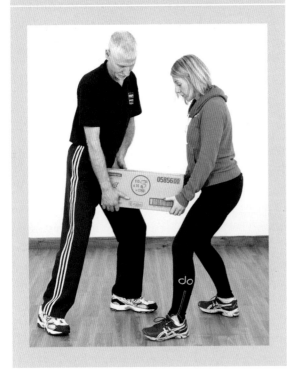

Purpose
To perform a squat lift action using a partner to lift a single heavy object.

Preparation
Begin facing your client, each with your feet hip-width apart with an object placed between you.

Action
Both of you should step forwards, each positioning your feet for a correct lift. Bend your knees to squat down towards the object ensuring that you both have the object close to your safe zones prior to lifting. Communicate the timing of the lift by counting '1-2-3 lift', and then '1-2-3 lower', to place the object back on the floor.

Tips
In order to lift correctly, each person must ensure that the object is positioned within their safe zone. It is essential that they walk their feet inwards rather than pulling the object towards themselves, and therefore away from their partner. Remember also that timing is vital.

PUSHING AND PULLING

Pushing and pulling actions involve the production of force with the legs, and the transmission of that force through the stable spine to the arms and hands as force appliers. One of the most common errors is trying to produce the power for the movement using the arms alone, or using the spine as a lever. We begin by practising force development in the horizontal direction using the legs, and then progress to continuous movements.

Exercise 8.8 Wall push

(a)

(b)

Purpose

To learn the correct body alignment for pushing during manual handling.

Preparation

Begin with your client facing a wall with their hands placed at mid-chest level, slightly wider than shoulder-width apart.

Action

The client steps backwards, lowering their hips slightly and straightening their arms, so that they form a relatively straight line from their hips through their shoulders to their hands. The client should bend their right knee and place their left foot back and press into the wall by pushing with their legs ensuring that their arms stay firm and their spine is correctly aligned.

Tips

The aim of this action is to generate force with the legs, transmitting the force through a stable spine and shoulders to apply force through the hands. Pushing power will be lost if the spine moves away from the neutral position into either flexion or extension, and if the elbows move apart or the shoulders lose alignment. The straighter the line from the feet through your hips and shoulders to the hands, the more direct the application of the force.

Exercise 8.9 Rope pull

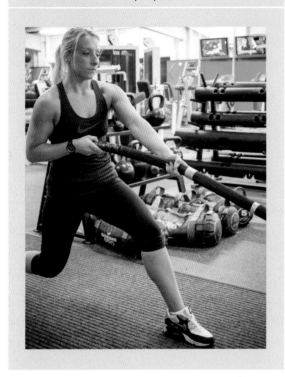

Tips

The power for the pulling action comes from the legs with the trunk leaning back to form a stable base. Both the knee and hip extensor muscles work in conjunction with the spinal extensors and shoulder adductors to create a powerful pulling action. Force is lost if the body alignment is poor or if core stability falters.

Purpose

To learn correct body alignment for a pulling action in manual handling.

Preparation

Begin holding a rope in both hands, standing with your feet hip-width apart.

Action

The client should straighten their arms and lean back, lowering their hips and bending their knees. They should press their feet into the ground, and draw their hands towards their chest holding their elbows in. Walk backwards timing each step so that you create a firm surface with your chest and shoulders as you pull.

Exercise 8.10 Bench push

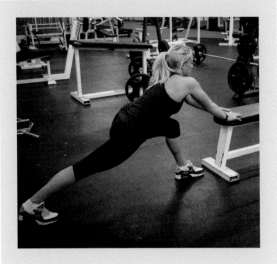

Purpose
To practise the coordination of pushing in a dynamic action.

Preparation
Your client should begin by standing at the end of a flat gym bench with feet hip-width apart. They step forwards with their left foot, bending their knees and sinking their hips down. They then place their hands on the edge of the gym bench, holding their hips low and aiming to form a straight line from their heels through their hips and shoulders to their hands.

Action
The client presses with their legs to drive their hips forward pushing through their straight arms onto the bench end, causing it to slide. They then gradually walk forwards, keeping their hips low and arms straight as they drive their legs down and back to create forward movement of the bench.

Tips
The power created from the legs is transmitted through the rest of your body. Power will be lost if alignment falters. Common errors include allowing the hips to raise upwards, flexing or extending the spine and allowing the elbows to drift outwards.

TORSIONAL ACTIONS
Torsion actions are especially important in unilateral (single-sided) actions which place more stress on one limb. Many injuries to the lower back, especially those involving the lumbar discs involve torsional activities, where the spinal discs undergo compression to the central nucleus and stretch to their annular casing. The aim of these next exercises is to restrengthen the muscles, creating torsional actions and supporting the spine, as well as rehearsing correct body alignment throughout torsional manual handling.

Exercise 8.11 High pulley twist

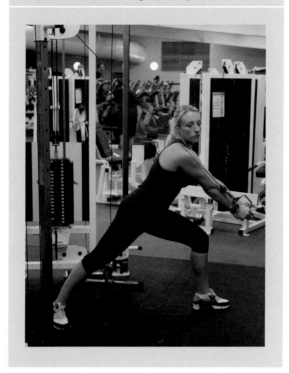

Action

The client keeps their arms locked and turns their body away from the machine, pulling the D ring downwards and towards them to reach past their far foot. They pause in the lower position and then unwind the movement slowly, turning towards the machine to lower the weight in a controlled fashion.

Tips

It is important during this exercise to maintain good trunk alignment, and not to move into marked spinal flexion or extension. The trunk rotator muscles create the force for movement and the knees can bend slightly (soften) to follow the movement. The force is created from the trunk muscles and transmitted through the locked arms. Some force will be lost if the arms bend.

Purpose

To work the trunk rotator muscles while maintaining correct whole-body alignment during a twisting action.

Preparation

The client begins by standing side-on to a height pulley with their feet shoulder-width apart. They should keep their hips facing forwards and turn their trunk towards the pulley machine. Instruct them to grip the D ring of the pulley in both hands.

Exercise 8.12 Low pulley twist (reverse woodchop)

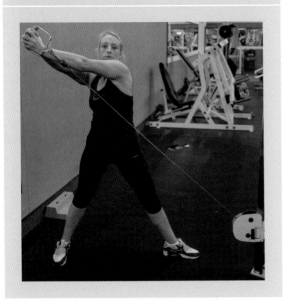

Purpose
To maintain good body alignment by creating a torsional force from a low starting position.

Preparation
Your client should begin standing side-on to a low pulley with their feet shoulder-width apart. Instruct them to bend their knees to reach downwards and grasp the handle of the low pulley apparatus, turning their chest to face the machine.

Action
Your client must pull the machine handle upwards and outwards, straightening their knees and turning their body away from the machine. They should keep their arms locked to transfer the power generated from their legs and trunk, pausing in the turned position and then lowering the machine under control, sinking down with their knees to replace the machine handle.

Tips
It is important during this exercise to maintain good trunk alignment and not to move into marked spinal flexion or extension. The trunk rotator muscles and legs create the force for movement, and it is transmitted through the locked arms. Force will be lost if the arms bend.

Exercise 8.13 Cross-body lift to shoulder

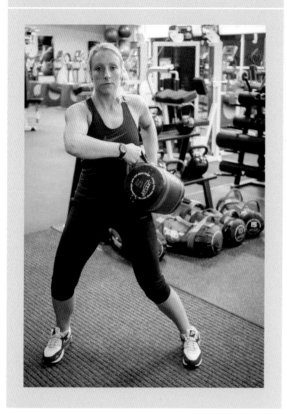

Action

Your client bends down, using leg and trunk flexion, combined with trunk rotation, and grips the medicine ball in both hands. They lift the ball straightening their legs and driving their body upwards to place the ball on their right shoulder. Pause in this position to readjust, allow the client to readjust their feet or trunk if needed, and then ask them to lower the ball back to the floor to their left side using a reverse action. Supervise five repetitions with the ball to the left followed by five repetitions with the ball to the right, in each case lifting to the opposite shoulder.

Tips

This action requires good timing to keep the ball close to the body line as it lifts, and the majority of force should come from the legs. Your client should keep the ball under control throughout the movement, not allowing momentum to build to such a degree that they lose control of the object.

Purpose

To use a diagonal movement pattern to perform a lift onto the shoulder.

Preparation

The client begins by standing with their feet shoulder-width apart, with a medicine ball or sandbag on the floor to their left.

Exercise 8.14 Overhead lift and twist

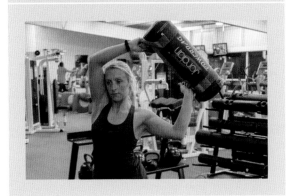

Purpose
To combine trunk movement and core stability with a functional overhead reach and lift action.

Preparation
Begin with your client holding a medicine ball or sandbag in both hands positioned to the side of their left thigh. Their trunk should be turned to the left to face their thigh.

Action
The client lifts the medicine ball upwards, and at the same time turns their trunk to face forwards. They keep the lifting action going until the medicine ball passes over their head, and then lower the ball while turning to their right. They then place the ball onto their right thigh to rest.

Tips
This exercise combines trunk movement while turning and trunk stability while lifting the object overhead. It is important to maintain good alignment and not hyperextend the spine during the lift. The object must be kept under control throughout the action as momentum can be high.

Exercise 8.15 Trunk rotation and lift

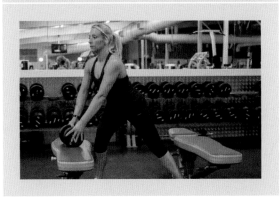

Purpose
To combine a repetitive lifting action with trunk rotation.

Preparation
Your client begins standing between two gym benches positioned approximately half a metre from each side of their body. Place a dumbbell on the bench to their right side; they should stand with their feet shoulder-width apart.

Action
Your client turns to their right, bending their legs and trunk, and lifting the object from the right side bench. They then draw the object in towards their safe zone at pelvis level, and turn to the left to place the object onto the left hand bench. Ensure they flex their trunk and legs to control the object's descent onto the bench.

Tips
Begin with a light dumbbell (5 to 10 kg) and increase the weight only when your client's technique is faultless.

Exercise 8.16 High pulley woodchop

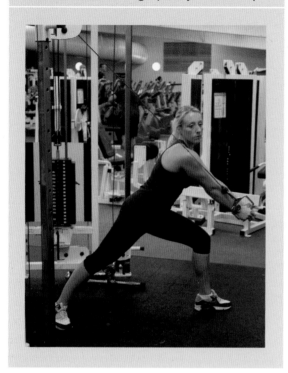

Action

Your client should draw the pulley handle downwards, at the same time rotating their trunk away from the pulley machine and bending their knees. They should then draw the pulley across their body to finish with it to the outside of their far knee. They should pause in this lower position and then reverse the action lowering the weight of the pulley under control as they rotate their trunk and allow their arms to raise back to the starting position. Instruct them to perform five repetitions facing in one direction and five facing the other.

Tips

As with all turning actions, momentum can build to high levels in this exercise. It is important to control the movement throughout the whole action and to pause in both the lower and upper positions at the end of each repetition.

Purpose

To combine a pulling and trunk rotation action.

Preparation

Begin with your client standing side-on to a high pulley with their feet shoulder-width apart. They should reach across their body to take hold of the handle of the pulley turning their body slightly to face towards the pulley machine.

YOGA FOR BACK REHABILITATION

9

A major systematic review of yoga for low back pain was conducted in Essen, Germany in 2013. The review looked at a total of 967 chronic low back pain patients over 10 scientific studies. The analysis showed that there was strong evidence for the short-term effects of yoga on pain, back-specific disability and global improvement. There was strong evidence for a long-term effect on pain and moderate evidence for a long-term effect on back-specific disability. This major study concluded that yoga can be recommended as an additional therapy to chronic low back pain patients (Cramer *et al*, 2013).

Definition

A systematic review is a scientific appraisal and summary of all the high-quality evidence available on a particular research question. It is one of the key components of evidence-based medicine (EBM), and is used to justify treatment selection.

Recent studies have shown yoga to be an effective tool in the management of low back pain. In a study looking at 313 adults with chronic low back pain, (Tilbrook *et al*, 2011), yoga was given as a 12-week programme and included postures, breathing exercises and guided relaxation. The yoga group recorded better back function at follow-up measured at three, six, and 12 months following intervention. A study of an intense one-week period of yoga for 80 chronic low back pain patients showed it to be superior to a physical exercise programme when spinal flexibility was measured (Tekur, *et al*, 2008). Yoga has been shown to be effective for war veterans with low back pain, improving pain, energy levels and mental health after a 10-week programme (Groessl *et al*, 2012). A randomised controlled trial (RCT) in the USA showed a 14-week yoga programme to give a clear improvement measured on a standard clinical research scale (Roland and Morris Disability Questionnaire or RMDQ) (Sherman *et al*, 2005) and a study which followed participants for 48 weeks shown improvement in functional disability measures, pain intensity and depression scores (Williams *et al*, 2009).

The evidence shows that yoga is an important intervention for low back pain, and significantly improves not just pain but mental and physical wellbeing. In chapter 4 we looked at the biopsychosocial nature of low back pain and saw that it was important to target not just the physical symptoms of the condition but the patient's belief systems as well. It would seem that yoga is an ideal therapeutic medium to attain this.

WHAT IS YOGA?

The term yoga means union (yoke) and refers to the union between body, mind, emotion and breath. Originally it is based on Hindu teaching, but nowadays a modified form of yoga, which falls into the category of mind-body exercise, is more commonly practised – often alongside activities such as Pilates, and Tai chi. Yoga can be seen as mindful activity in that it combines both physical exercise and a mindfulness approach to movement. Participants are encouraged to pay attention to the feeling of their body during exercise, with special attention to the breath. This concept of awareness of the breath is central to the mindfulness approach used in stress management (Williams and Penman, 2011). Classical yoga postures (asana) are linked to breath awareness and control (pranayama), concentration (dharana) and relaxation/meditation (dhyana).

Definition

Mindfulness is a psychological term inherited from the Buddhist tradition. It involves paying attention to the present moment in a non-judgemental way.

A typical yoga class begins with a centring activity designed to act as a buffer between the activities of daily living and the focus required in the yoga class. This would typically be a seated posture

Table 9.1	Common yoga styles
Style	**Emphasis**
Ashtanga	Individual posture combined into sequence. Emphasis on breathing as you move from posture to posture.
Iyengar	Posture, symmetry, and alignment. Props often used.
Sivananda	Traditional yoga with postures, breathing and meditation.
Hot yoga (Bikram)	Practised in heated room. Participants often wear swimwear due to sweating.
Fitness yoga	Fitness class using basic yoga postures as exercise types.
Power yoga	Modern version of Ashtanga yoga combining postures into moving sequence. Fitness based.

requiring the participant to close their eyes and focus on their breathing, for example, thus turning their attention inward towards their body and away from environmental stimuli. The body of the yoga class uses exercises typically practised on a non-slip (sticky) mat, and often uses basic props such as foam blocks, wooden bricks and webbing belts. Exercises are practised in a number of starting positions including lying, floor sitting, chair sitting, kneeling, and both free and wall support standing. Exercises are typically practised individually, but partner work can also be used. Yoga poses are normally taught within a class format but may be done on a one-to-one personal training basis. The speed of exercise and the amount of individual supervision varies depending on the yoga style taught. Table 9.1 lists some common yoga styles.

Typically a yoga class will involve several postures, progressing in intensity and finishing with a relaxation and/or meditation session. The postures are often held for a number of seconds and clients are encouraged to relax and breathe normally during the postures. Postures are normally practised symmetrically with emphasis on good alignment as well as range of motion. In addition, counter-poses are often used to prevent stress accumulation within the tissues. For example, postures emphasising spinal flexion are often countered by those emphasising extension. Body alignment when performing postures is usually compared to an idealised version typically presented by a yoga book, organisation or senior practitioner. Sometimes the reasoning behind the idealised postures lacks clear scientific evidence. Classical yoga usually claims that poses are passed down over the centuries from teacher to pupil, and many organisations claim to represent the true postures. Scientific scrutiny has challenged the claim of all yoga postures being ancient and the techniques unchanged over millennia (Singleton, 2010).

Table 9.2	Common yoga poses
Body part	**Animal**
• Pada: foot • Hasta: hand • Janu: knee • Sirsa: head • Mukha: face • Anga: limb • Bhuja: arm • Sarvanga: whole body • Sava: corpse	• Svana: dog • Bheka: frog • Baka: crow • Ustra: camel • Bhujanga: snake (serpent) • matsya: fish • Shalabha: locust (grasshopper)
Object	**Position**
• Parigha: gate latch • Hala: plough • Vrksa: tree • Tada: mountain • Setu: bridge • Nava: boat • Dhanu: bow • Danda: rod (staff) • Vira: hero	• Adho: downward • Urdva: raised/upward • Utthita: extended, stretched • Parivrtta: revolved • Baddha: tied/bound • Supta: reclining/sleeping • Uttana: intense stretch • Upavistha: seated • Prasarita: spread out • Ardha: half • Salamba: with support • Kona: angle

POSTURES FOR LOW BACK PAIN

Yoga postures (asanas) have individual names, which may describe the general body shape, an animal which the posture is supposed to resemble or an individual after whom the pose is named. Poses have both Western and Sanskrit names (see table 9.2), so for example Mountain pose is also called Tadasana, from the Sanskrit *Tada* meaning mountain and *asana* meaning posture.

Definition

Sanskrit is one of the original languages of the Indian subcontinent. Classical Sanskrit is rarely used nowadays except in traditional ceremonies in mainly Hindu and Buddhist practice. Versions of the language can be traced back to 1500 BCE.

Exercise 9.1 Mountain pose (*Tadasana*)

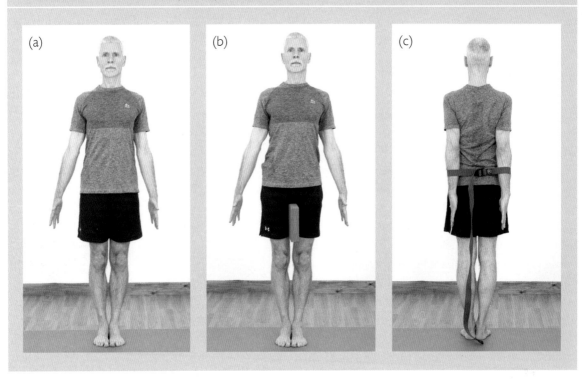

(a) (b) (c)

Purpose

Learning standing body alignment is a preparation for further poses, and to increase appreciation of optimal posture.

Preparation

The client begins standing with their feet together and hands by their sides, palms facing inwards.

Action

The client should take their weight equally between their right and left foot, and between the toe and heel on each foot. They should tighten their thigh muscles (quadriceps) to draw their knees straight and together. Tell your client to lengthen their spine reaching the crown of their head upwards and draw their shoulder blades together slightly to open their chest. They should then straighten their arms, reaching their fingertips downwards towards their outer ankle bones (lateral malleolus). Maintain the position breathing normally.

Tips

Some individuals hyperextend the knees when they tighten the quadriceps muscles. To avoid this action keep your client focused on maintaining a straight vertical line from their hips through their knees to their ankles. In addition they should avoid overarching their lumbar spine (hollow back posture) by gently drawing their abdominal muscles inwards and tailbone downwards.

Exercise 9.2 Triangle (*Trikonasana*)

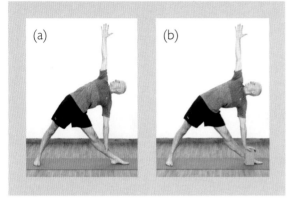

(a) (b)

Purpose

To lengthen the side trunk and outer hip.

Preparation

The client begins by standing on a yoga mat with their feet approximately one leg-length apart, toes facing forwards. They stretch their arms out sideways (shoulder adduction) keeping their elbows straight and palms facing the floor.

Action

Instruct your client to turn their left leg outwards (lateral rotation of the hip) so that their toes face the short edge of the mat. They should then reach their left hand out and downwards, placing it onto their left shin, while at the same time reaching their right hand upwards towards the ceiling. They should avoid allowing the right side of their pelvis to roll forward, and keep the pelvis aligned so that the hip joints are stacked (right and left joints aligned in a vertical position). They should open their chest and extend their thoracic spine into a light shoulder-retracted position. To come out of the pose the client reaches with their right arm upwards and presses with their left hand onto their shin. The action is then repeated on the right side of the body.

Your client should next perform a limited range action, taking the left hand down to a chair, placing their hand in the centre of the chair and keeping their arms straight. To increase range further, they may use a wooden yoga block placed with its long edge aligned vertically. The block should be aligned with the centre of the shin.

To improve alignment the action can be performed with the client's back towards the wall, while they try to press the upper pelvis backwards against the wall to maintain the stacked hip position.

To reduce balance demand, perform the standard pose, but keep your right hand on your hip, or place your hand behind your tailbone (sacrum) to encourage chest opening.

Tips

The triangle pose requires a combination of leg firmness and stability, with flexibility of the lateral trunk. The pose can be effectively split into two portions, practising leg stability with the hands on the hips initially. Once this has been attained the trunk movement and arm stretch may be practised.

Exercise 9.3 Warrior (*Virabhadrasana*)

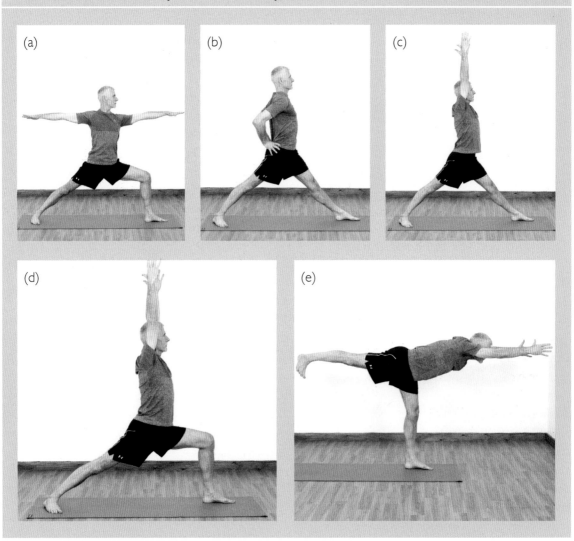

Purpose
To build leg strength while maintaining upper-body alignment.

Preparation
Your client should stand on a yoga mat with their feet wide apart (approximately half a leg length).

They should reach their hands out sideways so that their arms are straight, elbows locked, palms facing the floor.

Action
Instruct your client to bend their left knee, pressing it forwards over the left foot ensuring that it

does not drop inwards into a knock-knee position. This action should stop when the knee is at 90° and the shin is vertical, with the thigh horizontal. The client should press on the left foot to straighten their leg and draw back to standing. The movement is then reversed, bending the right leg. This pose is Warrior (II).

The client should lower their arms and place their hands onto their hips. They should turn their left leg outwards (outward rotation of the hip) to face their toes towards the short edge of the mat. Instruct them to turn their trunk to the left aiming to get their pelvis and shoulders facing the short edge of the mat. Bending their left knee, they press the knee over the left foot. They should stop when the knee is at 90° and their shin is vertical, thigh horizontal, then reach both arms overhead keeping them shoulder-width apart with their fingers straight and palms facing each other. Pressing on the left foot they should straighten their leg and draw back to standing, before reversing the movement by bending the right leg. This pose is Warrior (I).

After the final pose of Warrior (I), your client should lower their trunk towards their left thigh and step in with their right foot. They should press hard with their left leg and lift their leg into a horizontal position keeping their thigh muscles tight. Reaching forward with their hands, they should aim to form a straight horizontal line from their hands through their shoulders, trunk and right leg. Release the pose by reversing the action. This pose is Warrior (III).

Both Warrior (I) and Warrior (II) may be performed as limited range motion poses, bending the knee only as far as is comfortable. To provide additional support the left hand may be placed on a chair when moving to the left. As leg strength increases the knee may bend further until the 90° angle of the classical pose is obtained. Warrior (III) may be performed with the hands placed on a wall to aim balance and alignment.

Tips

There are two common errors which occur in the Warrior poses. The first is allowing the knee to drift inwards into a knock-knee position. This places extra stress on the inside (medial aspect) of the knee. To prevent this ensure that the knee passes over the centre of the foot. The second error is allowing the upper body to drop into a round-shouldered position which restricts the chest and breathing. Avoid this by ensuring your client lengthens their spine reaching the crown of the head upwards and keeping the chest open and the shoulders drawn back slightly.

Exercise 9.4 Wide legged forward bend (Prasarita Padottanasana)

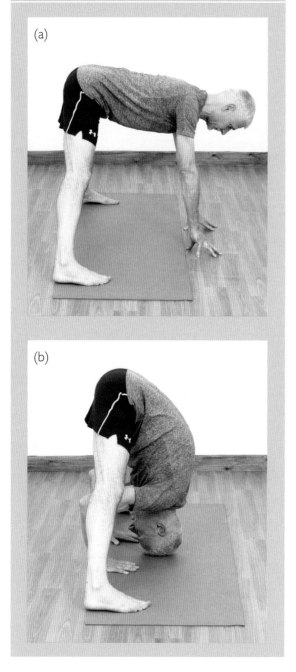

(a)

(b)

Purpose
To lengthen the hip tissues while maintaining lumbo-pelvic and upper body alignment.

Preparation
Begin with your client standing on a yoga mat with their legs apart, feet facing directly forwards.

Action
Your client should place their hands on their hips and fold their body forwards, keeping the spine straight and moving from their hip joints. When their trunk makes an angle of 90° to their legs, the client should place their hands on the mat directly beneath their shoulders.

To increase the intensity of the stretch, ask your client to bend their elbows and take their hands backwards to place them on the mat level with their feet. They should keep their spine as straight as possible aiming to place the crown of their head onto the floor.

To reduce the intensity of the pose get them to rest their forearms on the seat of a chair placed in front of them, or place their hands on to wooden yoga blocks placed shoulder-width apart on the mat in front of them.

Tips
As the trunk moves forwards there is a tendency for the spine to flex excessively. To avoid this the client should keep their hands on their hips and draw their elbows together to open their chest (retracting the shoulder blades and extending the thoracic spine). To further reduce this tendency the client may take their arms downwards, reaching and looking forwards to maintain the extension of the thoracic spine.

Exercise 9.5 Forward bend (*Uttanasana*)

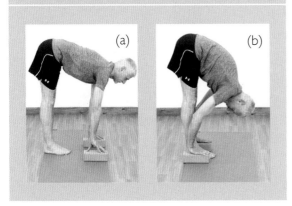

(a) (b)

Purpose
To lengthen the hamstring muscles, hips and spine from a standing position.

Preparation
The client begins by standing in mountain pose.

Action
The client should reach their arms forwards and then overhead, keeping their hands shoulder-width apart. They should angle their trunk forward, keeping their spine straight and arms reaching out in front to encourage thoracic spine extension. Reaching forwards and downwards they move their hands towards the floor. Placing their hands on the floor they should pause in this position, keeping the arms straight and thorax extended.

For the final pose, your client should reach their hands behind their heels and draw their trunk down onto their thighs. To come out of the pose they should release their hands from their heels and reach their arms forwards and upwards to extend their spine as they stand back in the upright position, before pausing in the mountain pose to recover.

To reduce the intensity of the stretch the client may reach their hands downwards onto wooden yoga blocks either placed on their long side (lower left) or short side (higher left). Where the hips are very stiff your client should begin the position with their feet shoulder-width apart, and where the hamstrings are very tight allow your client to bend their knees slightly (unlock or soften the knee) to partially release the pull of the hamstrings onto the pelvis and allow better lumbo-pelvic alignment.

Where standing balance is impaired the pose may be performed sitting on the edge of a chair. Position your client's sitting bones (ischial tuberosities) on the chair edge with the pubic bone slightly off the chair. Anteriorly tilt the pelvis, which will move the sitting bones backwards and then reach the arms forwards using gravity to increase the movement range.

Tips
This is an intense stretch to the hamstring muscles, and a high degree of hamstring flexibility is required to allow the pelvis to anteriorly tilt sufficiently to maintain spinal alignment. Where the hamstrings are very tight, anterior pelvic tilt is limited and downward movement can only be obtained by increasing spinal flexion. Where excessive spinal flexion occurs it is important to reduce the movement range and maintain good overall body alignment rather than sacrificing alignment simply to reach further towards the ankles.

Exercise 9.6 Staff pose (*Dandasana*)

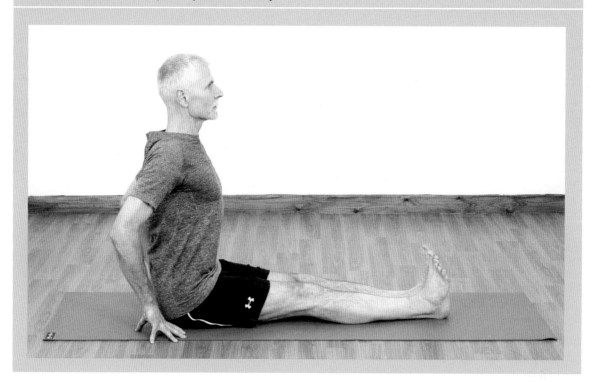

Purpose

To lengthen the hamstring muscles, and rehearse a correct straight leg sitting (long sitting) pose.

Preparation

Begin with your client sitting with their legs straight and spine upright. Their lumbar spine should be in its neutral position, with a gentle inward curve (lordosis).

Action

Have the client place their hands onto the mat on either side of their hips and press down gently to extend the thoracic spine and lift the rib cage (sternal lift action).

If they find it difficult to sit with their spine upright, ask them to sit with their back against a wall.

If the spine rounds in the sitting position, have them sit on one or two foam or yoga blocks to anteriorly tilt their pelvis and realign the spine.

Tips

It is often useful in this pose to act as your client's training partner. To encourage them, you can place the outside of your leg along the length of their spine, and gently draw their shoulders backwards pressing their spine into a straight position against your leg. The action is to encourage rather than force the movement, and you must ask your client to give feedback about what they are feeling in their back throughout the movement.

Exercise 9.7 Seated forward bend (*Paschimottanasana*)

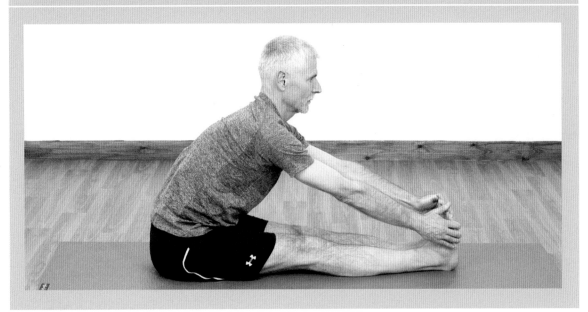

Purpose
To lengthen the hamstring muscles, hips and spine from a sitting position.

Preparation
The client should begin sitting in the staff pose, pressing their hands onto the floor to encourage thoracic extension and lifting of the ribcage.

Action
Your client reaches their hands forwards and then overhead, keeping their arms shoulder-width apart, to extend the thoracic spine. They should maintain this thoracic extension and then reach forwards towards their feet aiming to grasp their feet (knuckles outwards) and draw their upper body down onto their thighs.

Where the client is unable to reach their feet loop a yoga belt around their feet (place the belt in the middle of the sole to avoid it slipping). They should grasp the yoga belt with each hand and draw forwards aiming their lower ribs towards their thighs, rather than their head to their knees. To encourage lift in the ribcage encourage your client to move their elbows out to the side as they pull on the belt.

This action may also be performed sitting on a chair, changing sides where the pose becomes the same as the standing forward bend (Uttanasana) described above.

Tips
If the hamstring muscles are very tight, or your client has a tendency to hyperextend their knee, place a folded towel or yoga blanket beneath their knees. This will have the effect of bending the knee slightly (unlocking) to release the stretch in the hamstrings and tension in the posterior knee joint structures.

Exercise 9.8 Wide leg sitting (*Upavista Konasana*)

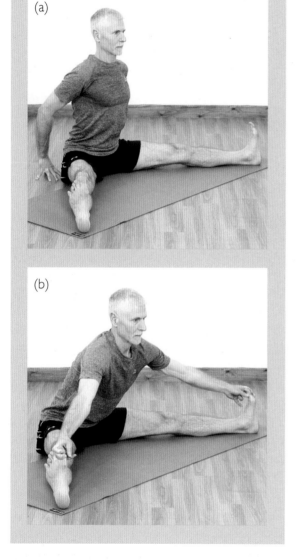

(a)

(b)

Preparation
Your client should begin in staff pose. If required they may sit on one or two yoga blocks to optimally align the pelvis and lumbar spine.

Action
Lift each leg in turn to the side (hip abduction) ensuring that they are equidistant from the body's mid-line. The toes must be kept pointing upwards, avoiding outward or inward rotation of the hip, and maintaining tension in the quadriceps muscles. Your client should press their hands onto the floor at the side of their body to open their chest and lengthen their spine.

Where the client finds it difficult to maintain spinal extension, use two yoga belts and loop them around the centre of each foot. The client can then hold one belt in each hand and gently pull on the belts, retracting the shoulders and lifting the sternum.

To provide further spinal support, the client may perform the exercise with their back pressed against a wall.

Tips
To ensure that their pelvis is correctly aligned, they should be sitting on their sitting bones (ischial tuberosities) and pubic bone. Where they have begun the pose with their pelvis posteriorly tilted, they should place one hand under each ischial tuberosity in turn and pull backwards drawing the buttock flesh (gluteal musculature) backwards.

Purpose
To lengthen the hamstrings and hip abductor muscles while maintaining an upright sitting posture.

Exercise 9.9 Seated twist (*Bharadvajasana*)

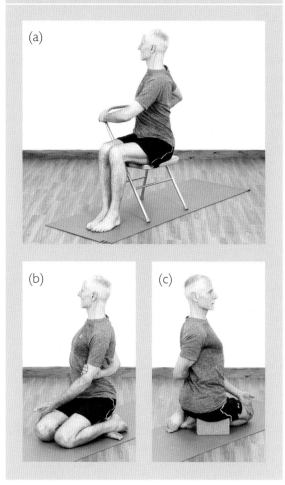

(a)

(b)

(c)

Action

Instruct your client to turn towards the chair back and grip the top of the frame in each hand, lifting their elbows away from the sides of their body and placing gentle overpressure to increase spinal rotation. Ensure that their shoulders remain horizontal throughout the action and they do not sideflex. Repeat the action facing in the opposite direction.

The client can perform the pose kneeling, with a folded towel blanket between their buttocks and heels to reduce the range of motion required at the knees. Get them to turn to the right, placing their left hand onto the side of their right knee, and their right hand behind them on the floor. They can then use their hands to encourage rotation range of motion and spinal lengthening.

Get them to perform the classical pose sitting on a foam yoga block, bending their left leg, placing their left foot to the outside of their left hip (hero or virasana pose leg position). They should bend their right leg, placing their right foot inside their right thigh so that it passes beneath their left shin (cobbler or baddha konasana pose position). Readjust the position of the yoga blocks so that their hips are aligned horizontally. They should now turn their trunk to the right, pressing their left hand against their right knee and placing their right hand on the floor behind them.

Purpose

To release spinal stiffness and increase mobility to rotation movement.

Preparation

Begin with the client sitting side-on to a yoga chair or firm dining chair. They should place their feet hip-width apart and flat on the floor, and sit upright to ensure spine alignment.

Tips

The aim of this exercise is to use overpressure from the arms to encourage a greater range of spinal rotation. It is common to be asymmetrical, with rotation being freer to one side than the other. With practice the motion range should become equal on both sides (i.e. it should be symmetrical) and increase.

Exercise 9.10 Legs up wall
(*Viparita Karani*)

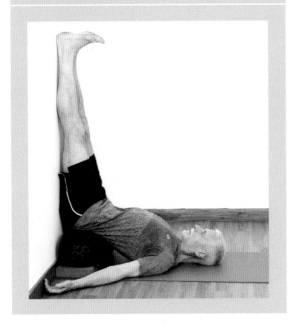

Tips
Your client's pelvis should rest on the raise, with enough room for their buttocks. If the buttocks alone rest on the yoga blocks this may feel insecure and you may find your client slowly creeps backwards as they relax. Placing the hips above the level of the chest reduces restriction in the abdominal region, and allows unrestricted diaphragmatic breathing. The height should be suitable for your client's body size.

Purpose
To rest the legs and increase lymphatic drainage and venous return.

Preparation
Begin by placing a yoga mat with its short edge against a wall. Stack yoga blocks or place a bolster against the wall, placed securely to avoid slipping.

Action
The client lies on their back with their knees bent and shuffles their hips forwards until their buttocks touch the wall, drawing their knees to their chest. They should extend their legs vertically against the wall, aiming to touch their buttocks, thighs and heels onto the wall surface. They should then relax in this position, breathing normally, for 2–3 min.

Exercise 9.11 Lying straight leg stretch (*Supta Padangusthasana*)

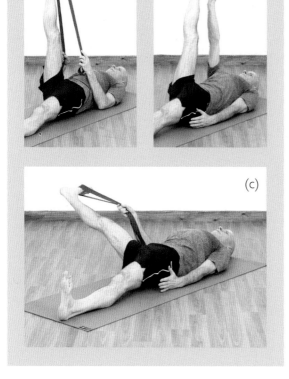

(a) (b) (c)

Purpose

To lengthen the hamstring muscles, sciatic nerve and posterior fascia of the leg.

Preparation

Begin with the client lying on a yoga mat on their back. They should draw their right knee towards their chest and loop a yoga belt around the sole of their right foot, holding each end of the belt in either hand.

Action

Keeping their left leg straight and pressed against the floor by tightening the quadriceps muscles, the client straightens their right leg by pressing the heel towards the ceiling keeping the knee over the hip. The client holds their leg in the vertical position for 10–20 seconds, breathing normally. They hold the belt, pressing their foot against it, and retract their shoulders to avoid flexing the thoracic spine.

Next they perform the previous action, and gradually draw their straight leg into further hip flexion by reaching their straight arms overhead, and at end range hold the position for 10–20 seconds, breathing normally. Repeat the action with the left leg.

Then ask your client to perform this action again, and transfer the belt to their right hand alone. They should draw their leg out sideways into adduction, keeping the foot in line with the hip. They may use their elbow against the floor as a point of contact. The aim is for them to take the side of their foot towards the floor to avoid external rotation of the hip.

Your client should now draw both knees towards their chest and loop a yoga belt around the soles of both feet, and straighten both legs pressing their heels towards the ceiling to create a 90° angle at their hips (classical Urdhva Parasite Padasana pose).

Tips

Each of these exercise sequences targets the posteriorly structures, with a different emphasis depending on the movement range and motion direction. Vary practice to ensure all structures are covered.

Exercise 9.12 Downward dog (*Adho Mukha Svanasana*)

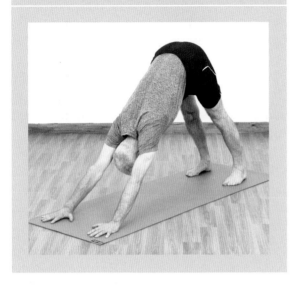

Tips

Where they find it difficult to press with their arms, place their hands onto yoga bricks positioned against the wall to avoid slippage. The heels of the hands should be at the front edge of the block to provide purchase. The higher block position encourages greater activity from the arms. Where they are unable to lower their heels to the ground place a block or folded blanket beneath their heels.

Purpose

To mobilise the chest, shoulders and hips.

Preparation

Begin with your client lying on their front on a yoga mat. Ask them to position their hands at the sides of their chest, with palms flat, and tuck their toes under tightening their quadriceps muscles to straighten their legs.

Action

Your client simultaneously presses with their hands and feet, driving their hips upwards. They should keep pushing until their arms are straight and level with their ears, and their hips are as high as possible. Instruct them to tighten their quadriceps and calf muscles, lifting high onto their toes. Maintaining this high pelvic position, they then gradually allow their heels to lower, placing a stretch on their calf and Achilles.

Exercise 9.13 Cobra (*Bhujangasana*)

(a)

(b)

Purpose

To increase spinal extension range of motion.

Preparation

Begin with the client lying on their front on a yoga mat with their feet together, and their hands at the side of their chest with the palms downwards.

Action

The exercise begins with the client retracting and depressing their shoulder blades, and extending their thoracic spine to gradually lift the breastbone (sternum) from the mat. Pressing with their arms to continue the movement, they should now extend their spine throughout its full length. Initially they should be looking in front, and then towards the ceiling (cervical extension). They should hold the upper position for three breaths and then lower under control.

Tips

The aim of this action is to move equally through the full length of the spine. As the thoracic spine is harder to extend than the lumbar spine there is a tendency to focus the entire movement in the lumbar area. To discourage this have your client visualise lengthening their tailbone and slightly posteriorly tilt their pelvis. However, ensure that the lower back and buttocks remain relaxed to reduce muscle tension in this area.

Exercise 9.14 Locust (*Salabhasana*)

(a)

(b)

Action

The client begins the action by tightening their thigh muscles and lengthening their legs, drawing their toes away from their head. The client should draw their fingers towards their heels and at the same time gradually lift their spine by coiling through its full length. Begin by asking them to draw their shoulder blades down and together (depression and retraction) and then lift firstly the upper and then lower portions of the breastbone (sternum).

Tips

There is a tendency with this movement to hyper-extend the lumbar spine restricting movement to one or two vertebral segments. To avoid this perform a minimal posterior pelvic tilt by encouraging your client to visualise lengthening their tailbone. The action should be slow and controlled avoiding any tendency to 'snap' the spine into extension.

Purpose

To strengthen the spinal and hip extensor muscles.

Preparation

Begin with the client lying on their front with their feet together and arms by their side, palms facing upwards.

Exercise 9.15 Plough (*Halasana*)

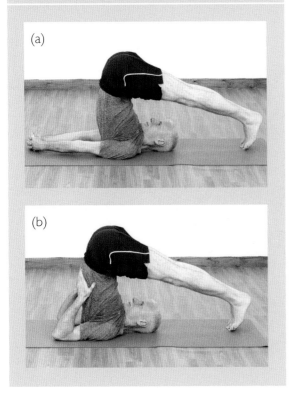

(a)

(b)

Purpose

To lengthen the posteriorly placed tissues and sciatic nerve.

Preparation

Begin with your client lying on their back with their hands by their sides, palms downwards.

Action

Instruct your client to draw their knees to their chest and press their hands onto the mat. They should continue the movement, rolling their spine into flexion. Allowing their legs to straighten, they should lock their knees and place their toes on the floor. They then bend their elbows to support their spine with their hands on their upper back. As they release the pose, they should draw their knees back into their chest and place their straight arms on the ground. They should finish by lowering their spine back onto the mat under control.

To reduce the range of motion, the client can place their toes on the seat of the chair rather than the floor. For additional support, they can place their shins on the chair seat padded with a folded blanket.

The range of motion can be reduced by performing the pose close to a wall, and resting the feet flat on the wall for support.

Your client can increase the workload on their shoulders by straightening their arms, interlacing their fingers, and pressing their straight arms downwards onto the floor.

Tips

This pose flexes the cervical spine significantly, placing stress onto the spinal tissues. To reduce flexion demands the pose can be performed with the shoulders on a pad. This can be four yoga blocks or two or three folded yoga blankets, of sufficient size for the shoulders to rest on and not slip over the edge. The head rests on the mat at a lower position than the shoulders, reducing the cervical flexion motion range.

Exercise 9.16 Inverted staff pose (*Viparita Dandasana*)

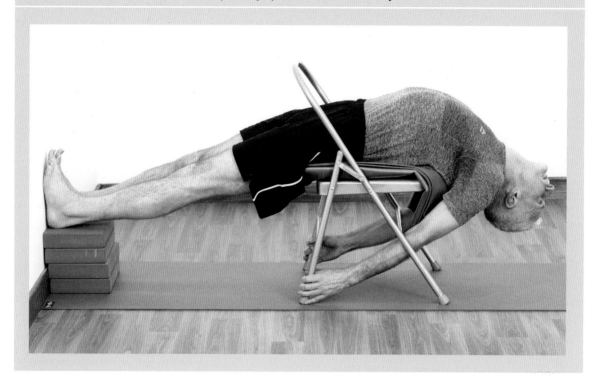

Purpose

To impart passive extension force onto the spine.

Preparation

Place a stack of yoga blocks against a wall, and have the client sit on a chair or gym bench placed leg length away from the wall.

Action

Lying supine on the chair seat with the feet flat on the floor, the client should shift their upper body up and down until the chair edge is in line with the lower part of their shoulder blade (inferior angle of scapula). The client should hold the chair frame for support and arch their spine backwards into extension over the chair seat edge.

They should then lift their feet one at a time onto the blocks and straighten their legs, tightening their quadriceps muscles and pressing their heels downwards onto the blocks.

The client should allow their head to lower downwards so the crown faces the floor, and reach their arms back and out to hold the lower frame of the chair.

To increase motion range, they may place their heels on the floor rather than on blocks.

Tips

This is an intense stretch for the spine, chest and shoulders. It is important to move into and out of the pose in a controlled fashion and to progress the exercise gradually as the range of motion allows.

Exercise 9.17 Bridge (*Setu Bandha*)

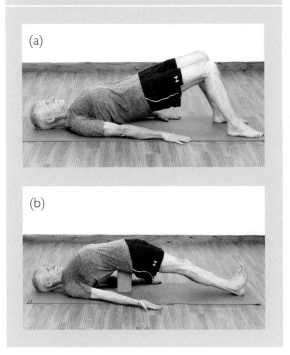

(a)

(b)

Purpose

To strengthen and mobilise the spine into extension.

Preparation

Begin with the client lying on their back with their knees bent and feet flat, arms by their sides, palms downwards.

Action

The client should press down with their hands and feet and lift their hips so that they form a straight line from their shoulders through their hips, thighs and knees. They should hold this position for three breaths and then slowly lower under control.

Instruct your client to perform the action again, and then bend their elbows placing their hands into their back on either side of the spine. The client should press with their hands to lift their chest. Once in the maximally lifted position, they should straighten first one leg and then the other, pressing their heels firmly into the ground and tightening their quadriceps muscles.

To reduce the work on the arms, the client may lift into the bridge position so you can place several foam blocks or a single wooden block (standing on end) beneath their pelvis. They should straighten their legs, tightening the quadriceps and pressing their heels firmly into the floor, keeping their arms on the floor at the side of their body, palms facing downwards.

Tips

Placing the hands or support further up the spine focuses the extension movement into the thoracic spine in addition to the lumbar spine. The action is an intense extension stretch and it will take time for the spine to release into this position. Build the height of the support gradually over several exercise periods. The pose should be challenging but not painful.

Exercise 9.18 Corpse pose (*Savasana*)

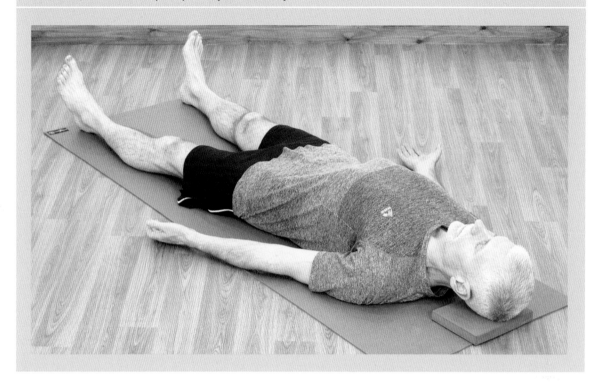

Purpose

To relax the body and aid recovery. The pose is often used for pranayama practice (see p. 197).

Preparation

Begin with the client lying on their back on a yoga mat.

Action

Adjust your client's alignment so that they have their feet apart, hands by their sides with palms facing the ceiling, lumbar spine released and in its neutral position. Their head should be central facing up towards the ceiling, eyes closed. Instruct your client to focus their attention on their breathing allowing their body to slowly relax. Identify any areas of tension by asking your client to try to release the muscles limb by limb.

Tips

Some clients find it very difficult to relax. To assist you should remove as much muscle tension as possible, by aligning the body optimally. Where the head is in a forwards posture (protracted) place a folded blanket behind it for support, and if the lordosis is very deep a rolled towel or blanket can be used for support. Sometimes placing a folded towel over the eyes helps to release tension and quieten the mind. Corpse pose is an exercise and as with any other requires progression in terms of holding time, and may take time for clients to get used to.

BREATHING EXERCISES

Breathing exercises in yoga are called Pranayama (from the Sanskrit words meaning extension of the breath or extension of life force) and we will look briefly at different types. Clinically the techniques have been shown useful in the management of stress/anxiety disorders and in the treatment of respiratory conditions. Looking at asthmatic patients, pranayama practised for 15 minutes twice daily for a two-week period has been shown to improve respiratory variables (forced expiratory volume, peak flow rate and inhaler usage) compared to control (Singh *et al*, 1990). Favourable respiratory changes (oxygen saturation) have also been shown in patients with chronic obstructive pulmonary disease (COPD) during a 30-minute yoga breathing session (Pomidori *et al*, 2009). Both yoga poses (yogasana) and yoga breathing (pranayama) have been shown to reduce stress levels by action on the HPA axis, increasing the effect of the parasympathetic nervous system (Sengupta, 2012).

The mechanics of breathing is covered in greater detail in other texts and we have seen in chapter 4 how the diaphragm is linked to the process of spinal stabilisation. There are four mechanisms

Table 9.3	Mechanics of breathing	
Types	**Movement**
• Diaphragmatic • Sternal • Lateral costal • Apical	• Diaphragm descends and abdominal wall relaxes • Sternum lifts forwards (pump handle action) • Ribs flare outwards (bucket handle action) • Top of ribcage & collar bones lift

involved in the breathing cycle (see Table 9.3) and pranayama aims to activate each.

As pranayama involves an expansion of the breath asanas are often used prior to pranayama practice to open the chest. Pranayama itself may be practised in sitting or lying, with a focus on keeping the chest open. If you have a client with a very round-shouldered posture it can be useful for them to sit against a wall and straighten their spine to expand their chest. When they are lying on their back in corpse pose fold a towel or yoga blanket lengthways and place it on the floor beneath their spine and ask your client to gently press their spine into extension and retract their shoulders.

BREATH AWARENESS

Initially it is important to make your client aware of their own breathing. They may practise in corpse pose, placing their hands on their abdomen to feel the abdominal wall move as they breathe, and then locating movement in the lower ribcage, sides of the ribcage, and upper ribcage. Once they are aware of these movements they

> ## Definition
> The HPA (hypothalamic-pituitary-adrenal) axis consists of a series of functional links between the hypothalamus (just above the brain stem), the pituitary, a pea-shaped gland located below the hypothalamus, and the adrenal gland sitting above the kidney. Each produces hormones which act on the other structures as part of stress and mood reactions.

should relax their arms onto the floor, close their eyes and focus their attention internally on these body movements.

EXPANSIVE BREATH (UJJAYI)

Expansive breath follows on from breath awareness and the student is encouraged to breathe in through their nose and out through their mouth, increasing the volume of the breath. The inhalation should be performed slowly and gradually without forcing or gulping air into the lungs. The abdomen is relaxed but not bloated, to allow the diaphragm to move unhindered. Aim to fill the lower (basal) part of the lungs by expanding the lower ribs, before the middle ribs and finally the upper ribs. Chest expansion should include lifting of the sternum (pump handle action), sideways and backwards expansion of the ribcage (bucket handle movement). Finally the top portion of the ribcage lifts (apical breathing).

As air passes over the roof of the palate it makes a rushing sound 'sssa', said to resemble an ocean, hence the alternative name of this pranayama: 'ocean breath'. If air is forced in rapidly it will rush over the palate causing throat irritation and coughing, so the action must be deliberate and controlled.

BELLOWS BREATH (BHASTRIKA)

Once your client has become aware of movement in the abdomen as a result of diaphragmatic breathing they can practise bellows breath. This is traditionally done in sitting and involves an inhalation followed by a sharp exhalation where the abdominal wall is tightened to force air out of the lungs rapidly. Three or four cycles are completed before practising normal breathing to recover. This recovery period is important to prevent dizziness due to hyperventilation.

INTERUPTED BREATH (VILOMA)

There are two stages to this technique. Firstly interrupted inhalation is used. The sequence is to inhale-pause-inhale-pause with each in-breath and pause lasting approximately two seconds. The breath is held at full inhalation for 3-5 seconds. The client exhales slowly but continuously and then breathes normally for 2–3 breaths to recover. In the interrupted exhalation the sequence is reversed. The client takes a single deep breath and holds it briefly before the interrupted exhalation cycle begins with the rhythm exhale–pause–exhale–pause with each period again lasting for two seconds.

ALTERNATE NOSTRIL BREATHING (NADI SODHANA OR ANULOMA VILOMA)

Many individuals have blocked sinuses, and it is typical for people to favour one nostril when they breathe normally throughout the day. Alternate nostril breathing helps to clear the sinuses and provide symmetry of breathing through all the nasal passages. In addition research has shown that there is alteration between right and left brain activity during this pranayama technique (Naveen et al, 1997). In the sitting position the client raises their right hand and places the thumb against the side of one nostril and the fourth and fifth fingers against the other, bending the middle and index fingers into the palm to allow room for the nose. The right nostril is blocked with the thumb as your client breathes in. They should pause while opening the right nostril and closing the left with the fourth and fifth fingers to exhale, pause and then reverse the technique. Between eight and ten breaths should be taken using this alternate nostril method before resting or breathing normally to recover. Commonly the breath is retained and exhalation increased, using a ratio of one to inhale, four to retain, and two to exhale.

RELAXATION & MEDITATION

Most yoga sessions finish with a period of relaxation, typically in the corpse pose. Relaxation can then naturally progress to forms of introductory meditation.

With the client in the corpse pose begin using a process of progressive relaxation. This involves repeatedly tightening (isometric contraction) and then releasing the muscles to induce a feeling of relaxation due to reduced muscle tone (post-isometric relaxation). The client begins by pointing and then pulling up the toes, followed by tightening the quadriceps muscles, hip adductors and gluteals. At each point they tighten the muscle firmly, hold the contraction briefly and then relax. Progress the sequence through the abdomen to the shoulders retracting the shoulder blades, straightening the arms to tighten the triceps and then forming a fist and straight finger action relaxing forearm and arm muscles. Finally encourage your client to frown, and then bite, to identify and release the facial and jaw muscles.

When the muscular sequences have been completed draw your client's attention to the general feeling of warmth throughout the muscles due to increased blood flow, and finish by bringing their attention to their breathing as a precursor to meditation.

Meditation is introduced by focusing the attention on an internal body rhythm, and breathing is most often used in a classical method called mindfulness of breathing (Anapanasati). Draw your client's attention to their breathing, encouraging them to notice movements in the abdomen and ribcage, and to feel the passage of the breath through the nostrils and over the top lip. Ask them to breathe in and then out and to count one out loud, then repeat this action, counting two on the second breath and counting three on the third breath until they have completed 10 breaths. The sequence is then repeated. This action creates a deliberate pause after exhalation, as well as focusing the mind on the breathing sequence. Secondly, change the order, counting *before* they take a breath. This method again inserts a deliberate pause, this time prior to inspiration. Having mastered this technique they continue counting the breath in their mind, before progressing to simply noticing the passage of the breath through the nostrils and upper lip. It is normal for the attention to wander, and they can return to the counting method to draw their attention back within themselves once more.

FURTHER READING

Iyengar, B. K. S. (2001) *Light on yoga* (Thorsons, London).

Mehta, S. (1990) *Yoga: the Iyengar way* (Dorling Kindersley, London).

Sivananda yoga centre (2000) *The new book of yoga* (Ebury Press, London).

Trewhela, A., and Semlyen A. (2011) *Yoga for healthy lower backs* (Lotus Publishing, Chichester).

CLINICAL PILATES FOR BACK REHABILITATION

10

Pilates is a method of exercise instruction whose popularity closely parallels the use of core stability in the rehabilitation of low back pain. Pilates was originally developed by Joseph Pilates in the 1920s, and evolved over a number of years. Although the title Pilates derives from the inventor's name, it is considered a generic term for an exercise form (similar to yoga or weight training for example) following an intellectual property lawsuit in America in 2000 (www.pilates.com accessed July 2013). Pilates wrote two books: *Your Health* (1934) and *Return to Life through Contrology* (1945), both republished as collectors' editions in 1998. Pilates himself died in 1967, but his wife Clara and his former students continued to teach his methods, largely in America, based from their New York studio. The technique was used in the 1960s in the UK, but was mainly confined to the rehabilitation of dancers. The original techniques were modified and developed into a more widely available fitness form in the 1980s, and several organisations now teach the techniques. The exercises used will be familiar to any therapist using core stability work, but the methods of instruction differ to those traditionally used within physiotherapy. Pilates is often used as small-group work, or taught one-to-one,

and equipment is frequently used. Matwork is probably the most widely known form of Pilates.

The popularity of Pilates both for fitness and within the rehabilitation field has led to a considerable body of research looking at its effectiveness in the management of low back pain, and comparing it to other forms of rehabilitation. A recent systematic review (Wells, 2013) identified 44 reviews using the search terms of 'Pilates', 'review' and 'low back pain'. Of these, five systematic reviews were deemed to be of leading quality and are listed in table 10.1. All reviews argued that often the research quality of studies was poor, evidence inconclusive and that further research was warranted. Clear evidence was shown, however, for the benefit of Pilates in the management of low back pain.

FEATURES OF THE PILATES METHOD

Pilates exercise uses a number of key elements, which are used in each exercise. These were originally described as six principles (see table 10.2), but with the advent of research into areas of posture and core training these principles are interpreted and emphasised differently by different teaching organisations (Lawrence, 2008).

Table 10.1	Systematic reviews of Pilates method
Study reference	**Quoted results**
La Touche R, Escalante K, Linares MT: Treating non-specific chronic low back pain through the Pilates Method. J Bodyw Mov Ther 2008, 12:364-37.	All studies analysed demonstrated positive effects, such as improved general function and reduction in pain when applying the Pilates Method in treating non-specific CLBP in adults.
Lim ECW, Poh RLC, Low AY, Wong WP: Effects of Pilates-based exercises on pain and disability in individuals with persistent non specific low back pain: A systematic review with meta-analysis. J Orthop Sports Phys Ther 2011, 41:70-80.	Pilates-based exercises are superior to minimal intervention for pain relief. Existing evidence does not establish superiority of Pilates-based exercise to other forms of exercise to reduce pain and disability for patients with persistent non-specific low back pain.
Pereira LM, Obara K, Dias JM, Menacho MO, Guariglia DA, Schiavoni D, Pereira HM, Cardoso JR: Comparing the Pilates method with no exercise or lumbar stabilisation for pain and functionality in patients with chronic low back pain: Systematic review and meta-analysis. Clin Rehabil 2012, 26:10-20.	The Pilates method did not improve functionality and pain in patients who have low back pain when compared with control and lumbar stabilisation exercise groups.
Posadzki P, Lizis P, Hagner-Derengowska M: Pilates for low back pain: A systematic review. Complement Ther Clin Pract 2011, 17:85-89.	Some evidence supporting the effectiveness of Pilates in the management of low back pain.
Aladro-Gonzalvo AR, Araya-Vargas GA, Machado-Diaz M, Salazar-Rojas W: Pilates-based exercise for persistent, non specific low back pain and associated functional disability: A meta-analysis with meta-regression. J Bodyw Mov Ther 2012.	Pilates was moderately superior to another physiotherapy treatment in reducing disability but not for pain relief. Pilates provided moderate to superior pain relief compared to medical intervention and a similar decrease in disability.

Source: Wells *et al* (2013).

Pilates was originally termed contrology, and this perhaps illustrates one of the fundamental principles of the Pilates method: that movements are controlled. Ballistic actions and momentum are not typically used: instead every aspect of an action (start, middle and end) is controlled rather than haphazard. Together with yoga (described in chapter 9), Pilates is a mind/body exercise and encourages clients to develop a mindful approach (a term originally called concentration) to exercise is important. Many exercise programmes are performed nowadays with little self-focus. For example, somebody may exercise in a commercial gym watching television, or listening to music,

Table 10.2	Principles of Pilates teaching
Principle	**Practical method**
Control	Movement practised without momentum. Focus on start, execution and finish of exercise, controlling each aspect of an exercise.
Concentration	Developing mindfulness or focus of the body on items such as body part positions, muscle tension, breathing, instability and facial expression.
Centring	Engaging the muscles, stabilising the centre of the body (axial skeleton) by using the muscle stabilising the lumbar, scapular, cervical stabilisers and hip regions. Central body region termed the 'powerhouse' in traditional Pilates.
Precision	Optimising body alignment by considering neutral spine position, scapular alignment, pelvic position, ribcage position and limb alignment.
Breath	Differentiate diaphragmatic, ribcage and apical breathing actions. Focus on expansion of ribcage laterally as well as anteroposteriorly. Generally breathe out when chest is compressed by body flexion, or on effort. Breathe in with limb extension or as chest opens.
Flowing movement	Continuous fluid movement with correct timing between movement initiation (concentric), holding (isometric) and limb lowering (eccentric). Smooth transitions between portions of a movement, to produce a smooth effortless action.

Source: Ferris, 2013.

both approaches taking the client's attention away from their body. A mindful approach throws the focus back onto the body to foster awareness of things such as the position of one body part relative to another, tone (tension) within a muscle, breathing and the stability of one body segment relative to the moving limb.

Body alignment is central to the Pilates approach, and whole-body as well as body-segment alignment is important to the precision of a movement. Whole-body alignment is related to the starting position selected, while body-segment alignment is an awareness of the position

of one element of the body in relation to another during movement (in therapy terms this is known as 'segmental control'). The aim with Pilates is to remove uncontrolled aspects of a movement and refine the action to a precise, accurate, skilled action.

Clients often hold their breath when performing a new exercise which demands attention, and may breathe too deeply on exercises where resistance is used. The concept of breath awareness is important to Pilates (as with yoga) and the breath should flow freely with activity in all areas of the lungs. Often clients restrict their breathing to the apical section of the ribcage, due to tightness of clothing and postures taken up by positions at an office desk or when driving. Pilates offers an opportunity to re-educate breathing and make the client aware of diaphragmatic, costal and sternal breath movements. Where an exercise is more intense the general advice is to breathe out during the effort portion of the exercise (or where an action compresses the ribcage through trunk flexion), and in for recovery. If clients find breath timing of this type difficult to coordinate, simply allowing the breath to flow unhindered is sufficient in most circumstances.

'Centring' is one of the original concepts of Pilates, in modern terms this means engaging the core muscles. It is the understanding that for the limbs to move efficiently the central part of the body must remain firm to provide a stable base for movement. The early stage exercises covered in chapter 6 are particularly relevant here. Pilates has several useful methods of cueing and visualisation, which make learning voluntary contraction of the deep abdominal muscles and control of pelvic tilt easier. Visualisations, such as imagining that you are wearing a tight pair of jeans and zipping up the abdominal muscles as you put the jeans on, can be useful. A useful visualisation for contraction of the pelvic floor muscles is the pelvic elevator. In a sitting position the pelvic floor muscles can be drawn upwards as though there were an elevator in the groin. Floors of the elevator can be used to control muscle intensity, pulling the pelvic elevator to floor two or three to give 30 per cent voluntary contraction, while floor eight or nine would involve 80 per cent voluntary contraction.

When lying on the floor in a neutral position, we engage the deep abdominals and pelvic floor (local muscle system or LMS). Contraction of the

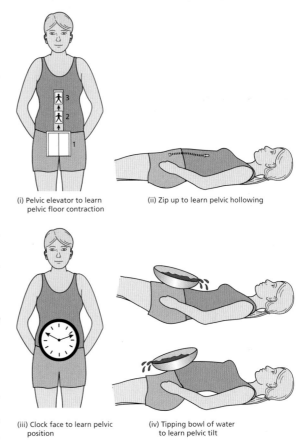

(i) Pelvic elevator to learn pelvic floor contraction

(ii) Zip up to learn pelvic hollowing

(iii) Clock face to learn pelvic position

(iv) Tipping bowl of water to learn pelvic tilt

Figure 10.1 Visualisations for improving abdominal muscle control

superficial abdominals (global muscle system or GMS) prior to performing an exercise will press the lower back gently towards the floor. It should make only light contact, and give a feeling of sliding the ribcage downwards (ribcage depression) a position called 'imprint'.

Imagining a source of water placed on your abdomen when you are lying on your back can be a useful visualisation for control of pelvic position. Tilting the pelvis to tip water from the top of the source gives posterior pelvic tilt, while pouring water from the bottom of the source gives anterior pelvic tilt. Imagining the umbilicus as the centre of a clock and using 12 o'clock, 6 o'clock, 3 o'clock

Table 10.3	Pilates terminology
Position	**Definition**
Tabletop	Starting position lying on the back with knees and hips bent to 90° so that the thigh (femur) is perpendicular to the floor and the shin (tibia) is parallel to the floor.
Imprint	Starting position lying on the back with deep abdominal muscles (local stabilisers) engaged, followed by minimal activity of the superficial abdominals (global stabilisers) to press the lumbar spine towards the floor to give very light contact only.
Neutral	Depth of lumbar lordosis created by pelvic tilt midway between full available posterior tilt (flatback) and full available anterior tilt (hollow back).
Chin tuck	Upper cervical flexion to engage the cervical stabilising muscles and flatten the cervical lordosis slightly. Also called head nod.
Stacked	One body part directly above the other. Typically used for vertebrae.
Soft	Joint just short of full extension. Typically used for the knee in standing, and the elbow in all fours position.
Navel to spine	Abdominal hollowing where the umbilicus is drawn inwards by action of the deep abdominal muscles. Breath should be unrestricted.
C-curve	Maintaining flexion throughout the whole length of the spine. Involves chin tuck, thoracic and lumber flexion and posterior pelvic tilt.
J-curve	Flexion of the upper portion of the spine (cervical and thoracic regions) only.
Domed abdominals	Imbalanced activity of the superficial abdominals compared to the deep abdominals causing the abdominal wall to bulge outwards (dome) during contraction.
Powerhouse	Area between the lower ribs and pubic bone. Working the powerhouse involves contraction of the deep abdominals, pelvic floor and hip musculature. Term inherited from Eastern medical systems where there are said to be energy centres in this region.
Smile muscles	Lower portion of the gluteus maximus at the point where the gluteal fold contacts the hamstrings. Used to emphasise pulling the gluteals in and upwards with contraction.
Sitting bones	Ischial tuberosities.

and 9 o'clock as positions to move the pelvis is again a useful visualisation.

Pilates exercises are said to be flowing movements, in that they focus on each stage of an action but do not stop or allow breath holding.

Ultimately, with practice, actions appear effortless and natural, like the performance of a skilled dancer or skater. Each movement changes to another (the change being termed a transition), in a smooth, refined way.

Exercise 10.1 Standing bodysway

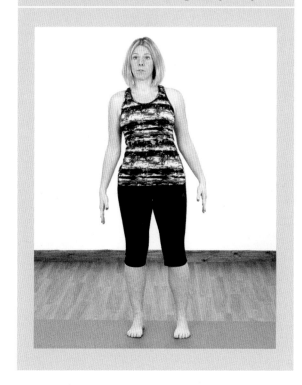

hip-width apart and knees just short of full extension, and their hands by their sides.

Action

Your client should sway their bodyweight forwards towards their toes, and then backwards towards their heels (this is called a 'toe-heel sway'). They stop in the mid-position when they have weight equally distributed between toes and heels.

Instruct your client to sway their bodyweight from side to side, taking more into their right leg and then more into their left (this is called 'side sway'). Stop them in the mid-position when they have equal weight distributed between both feet. Increase their awareness of their bodyweight through foot contact on the floor, ensuring that it is taken evenly between right and left leg, and toes and heels.

Tips

It is common, in the swayback posture, to favour the dominant leg, and take 80 per cent of the bodyweight through this leg, leaving only 20 per cent through the opposite side. The aim of this exercise is to increase awareness of weight distribution so that there is some overflow into day-to-day activities to improve postural awareness and postural control.

Purpose

To increase awareness of standing body position, and body weight distribution.

Preparation

Begin with your client standing with their feet

Exercise 10.2 Standing foot pedals

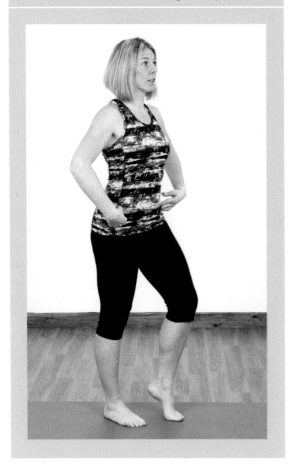

Action

Your client should shift their bodyweight to their left, and lift their right heel, raising onto the toes of their right foot. They should then lower their right heel, transfer their bodyweight to their right, and lift their left heel, raising onto the toes of their left foot. They continue the movement, alternately raising and lowering the heel on each leg, keeping their pelvis horizontal as they transfer bodyweight from foot to foot. Body sway should be kept at the minimal level required to perform the action accurately.

Tips

Begin this action slowly, focusing their attention on the accuracy of the horizontal pelvic movement. Once accuracy has been obtained, speed the movement up to become a rhythmic but flowing side-to-side action.

Purpose

To optimise side-to-side weight transfer during standing leg movement.

Preparation

Begin using standing bodysway to ensure that your client's bodyweight is evenly distributed over both feet.

Exercise 10.3 Standing spinal twist

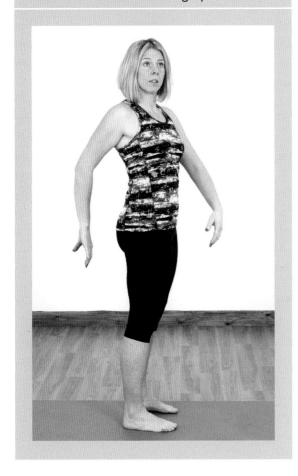

Purpose

To perform a spinal twist, isolating the movement from the hips.

Preparation

Begin with the client standing with their feet hip-width apart and bodyweight evenly distributed.

Action

The client should keep their hips facing forwards and slowly turn their spine to the right, moving their left hand in front of them and their right hand behind. Instruct them to pause at the full range position and then reverse the exercise, moving back to the centre and then to the left, taking their right hand in front of them and their left hand behind.

Next, the client should stand with their feet hip-width apart, arms extended out to their sides, palms facing forwards. They turn their spine to the right, maintaining the relative composition to that of their trunk, pausing at the full range position and then reversing the action, returning to the start, and then turning to the left.

From the standing position, they raise their arms forwards to the horizontal, palms facing each other. Ask them to turn their trunk to the right, bending their elbow and drawing their right hand backwards and reaching their left straight arm forwards. They should pause at end range and then reverse the movement, reaching the right arm forwards and bending their left.

Tips

The action should be a rotation through the full length of the spine, moving vertebra by vertebra, avoiding excessive movement in one area and stiffness in another. The head and neck should follow the movement rather than leading it.

Exercise 10.4 Monkey squat

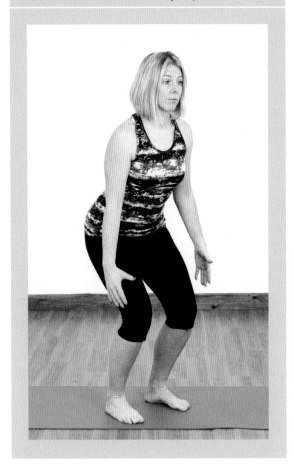

Purpose

To improve lumbo-pelvic rhythm in a freestanding posture.

Preparation

Begin with the client standing with their feet slightly wider than hip-width apart and parallel or very slightly turned out (10–15° external rotation of hip). Their hands are positioned at the sides of the thighs, or resting on the thighs for support.

Action

Ask the client to inhale, and as they exhale bend their knees and angle their trunk forwards (hip hinge action), sliding their hands down the front of their thighs towards their knees. Pause when their hands are at mid-thigh level and tell them to inhale to return to the starting position.

They should then place their hands by their sides, and bend their knees angling their trunk forwards. As they lower their body they should raise their arms to a horizontal position, turning their palms inwards so that their thumb leads the movement. Pause in the quarter squat position with their arms lowered (as pictured), and then tell them to raise, reversing the movement to lower their arms back to their sides.

Tips

Throughout this action your client should maintain a neutral lumbar spine position performing the trunk tip using an anterior pelvic tilt. As their shoulders move forwards their hips must move backwards to balance their bodyweight, and a useful visualisation is to imagine that they are perching on a high stool. The action of the hips should be essentially downwards with this small of amount of backwards movement only. They should avoid thrusting their hips too far backwards and moving their trunk into a more horizontal position.

Exercise 10.5 Standing roll down

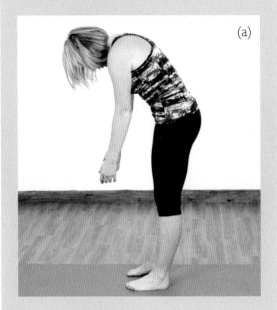

(a)

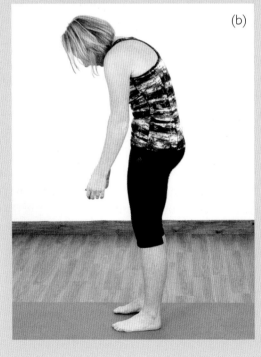

(b)

Purpose

To isolate spinal movement from pelvic movement in the standing posture.

Preparation

Begin with the client in a standing posture with their feet hip-width apart, hands by their sides.

Action

The client bends forwards, moving from the spine, vertebra by vertebra, initiating the movement from their neck and thoracic spine. Pause when their hands reach mid-thigh level and then ask them to roll their spine back up again, moving vertebra by vertebra (partial roll down).

The client should perform the partial roll down as above, and continue the movement, reaching their arms down towards the floor, allowing their pelvis to tilt as they do so. They should aim to move throughout their whole spine vertebra by vertebra, keeping their body close to the legs. They should now pause at full range without straining, and then reverse the movement, rolling back up leading with the posteriorly pelvic tilt followed by spinal extension (full roll down).

Tips

The forward bending action combines both anterior pelvic tilt and spinal flexion to perform a coordinated lumbo-pelvic rhythm. The partial roll down emphasises the spinal portion of the movement while the full roll down brings in pelvic tilt. The partial roll down may also be practised with the back against a wall, feet slightly forwards. The wall gives feedback (tactile cueing) about the upright position. The aim of the full roll down is to perform a smooth movement throughout the whole spine and pelvis.

Exercise 10.6 Lying single leg circle

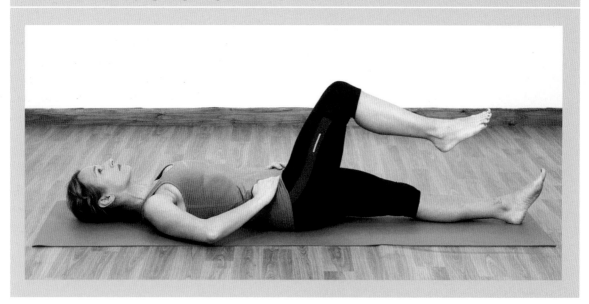

Purpose
To maintain a stable core while imposing overload due to leg movement.

Preparation
Begin with your client lying on their back with their knees bent, feet flat (crook lying).

Action
The client lifts their right foot by flexing their hip until their thigh is vertical, knee flexed (tabletop position). They should circle their knee first one way and then the other, keeping their trunk stable and immobile.

They should maintain gentle pressure of their lumbar spine towards the ground (imprint) and should not allow their abdominal wall to balloon, instead maintaining a single flat surface.

They should perform action number 2 and straighten the leg, describing circles with the straight leg and maintaining the neutral position of the lumbar spine.

Tips
In each of these exercises the position of the trunk is maintained as the stable base upon which the leg moves. To take some of the weight of the leg place a belt around the back of the thigh and hold the belt in each hand. It is common to notice that one hip is stiffer than the other, and this exercise acts both as a hip mobilising movement and an opportunity to enhance control of two body segments: hip and trunk.

Exercise 10.7 Seated spinal twist (Cossack)

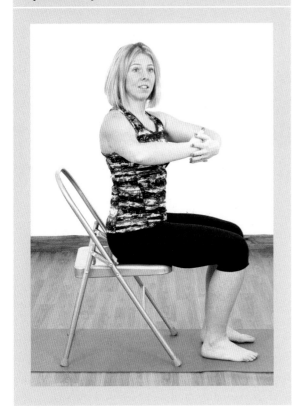

Purpose
To mobilise the spine to rotation while maintaining optimal spinal alignment.

Preparation
Begin with the client sitting on a firm chair or gym bench with their hips and knees at a 90° angle, feet flat. The client should loosely fold their arms, placing their hands together and keeping their upper arms at shoulder height.

Action
Instruct your client to lengthen their spine, positioning their lower back into its neutral position. They should activate their abdominal muscles (centring) and turn to their right, keeping their head in line with their breastbone (sternum), before pausing at the full range position and then returning to the start, repeating the action, turning to the left.

To increase the feeling of chest opening (shoulder retraction and sternal lift), place a pole across your client's shoulders and ask them to lightly grip it with their hands double shoulder-width apart. Have them perform the same rotation movement, using the pole to place overpressure on the spine to increase motion range.

Tips
The action is controlled throughout range by muscle contraction rather than momentum, and there should be no bouncing at end range. It is common for one side to be more flexible than the other (asymmetry). Continue the action with the aim of re-establishing symmetry.

Exercise 10.8 Swimming from lying

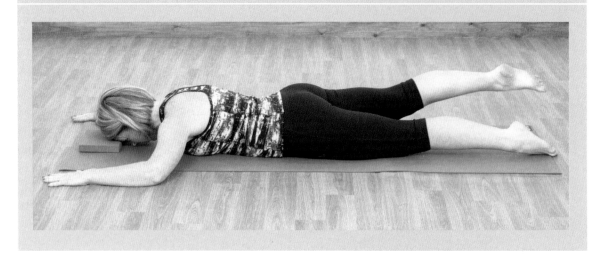

Purpose

To strengthen the shoulder retractor, hip extensor and spinal extensor muscles in prone lying.

Preparation

Begin with the client lying on their front with a folded towel beneath their forehead. They should then hold their arms slightly adducted and bent at the elbows to draw their hands to shoulder level ('W' position).

Action

The client engages their core muscles to maintain the neutral position of the spine (centring). Stretching their right leg, they reach it backwards and upwards, tightening their gluteal muscles as they do so. They should pause in the upper position before lowering the leg, repeating the movement on their left side.

Next, instruct them to retract and depress their shoulders to stabilise their scapula position. They should lift their right arm 5 cm from the floor and

straighten it, reaching their fingers forward to give the feeling of lengthening their arm. They pause in this outward position before lowering, and repeating the action on the left side.

Combine the two actions, with your client lifting their opposite arm and leg, raising their left leg and right arm, returning to the rest position and then raising their right leg and left arm.

Tips

The arm and leg raise from the floor only a small distance, so spinal alignment is maintained. The head can remain on the folded towel to support the neck. Avoid any hyperextension action in the spine by keeping the core muscles engaged and lifting the limbs to a low position only. As they lift their opposite arm and leg, suggest to your client that they visualise a piece of string attached from their fingertips to the tips of their toes. As they perform the exercise, they should visualise stretching the string to gain length in their limbs.

Exercise 10.9 Scissors

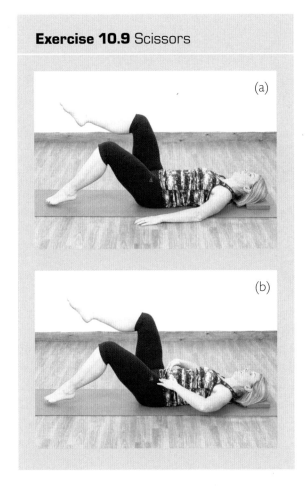

(a)

(b)

Purpose

To strengthen the core stabilising musculature and hips from a spine-supported lying position.

Preparation

Begin with the client lying on their back with their hips flexed to 90° and their knees bent, arms reaching upwards towards the ceiling (tabletop position).

Action

Your client inhales and keeps their arms reaching upwards, exhales extending their right hip to lower their foot towards the floor, maintaining the 90° angle at the knee. They should touch the floor briefly and then inhale to draw their leg back to the starting position, maintaining the neutral body position throughout the action.

Make the action easier (regress) by beginning with the client's legs in the tabletop position, and allow their knees to bend further so their heel moves towards their buttocks (short lever arm). The client should place their hands by their sides, palms downwards (support). As before, they lower one foot towards the floor, touch and then return to the start.

Next the client begins with their legs and arms in the tabletop position, maintaining the 90° angle at the knee. They lower their right leg to touch the foot onto the floor, as they lift the right leg back up, they lower their left leg to form a continuous scissor action with both legs.

Finally begin with your client's legs and arms in the tabletop position, and have them lower their bent right knee towards the floor and at the same time reach their straight left arm overhead. Pause when their foot and hand make contact with the floor, then draw the limbs back into the starting position and repeat the action, lowering the left leg and right arm.

Tips

Actions 3 and 4 are quite intense. Remind your client to breathe throughout the actions and avoid holding their breath.

Exercise 10.10 Dart

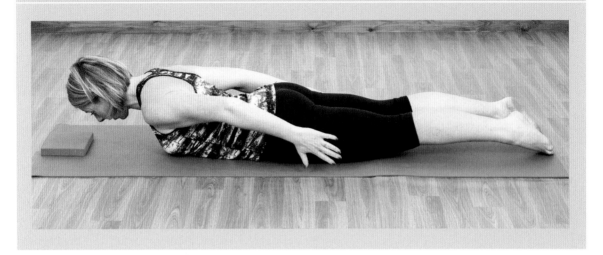

Purpose

To build endurance of the shoulder retractors and spinal extensor muscles.

Preparation

Begin with the client lying on their front on a gym mat with a folded towel placed beneath their forehead. Ask them to hold their arms by their sides, palms facing inwards.

Action

Your client should perform a scapular squeeze action by drawing their shoulder blades down (depression) and together (retraction). Lifting their arms off the ground, they should keep their head on the floor.

Have your client perform the scapular squeeze and arm lift as above, and lift their trunk into minimal extension so their head and upper breastbone (sternum) clear the floor, but their lower sternum stays on the floor.

Tips

The aim of this action is to maintain length of the body. The sensation should be of drawing the crown of the head along the ground as the trunk is lifted. The action of reaching the fingers towards the outer ankle encourages shoulder depression.

Key point

The scapula is attached to the ribcage by muscles alone, and does not make any bony connection. The two most important scapular stabilising muscles (those which hold the scapula onto the ribcage firmly) are the serratus anterior and the lower fibres of the trapezius muscle. Their combined action is to draw the scapulae flat onto the ribcage, and slightly downwards.

Exercise 10.11 Kneeling cat paws

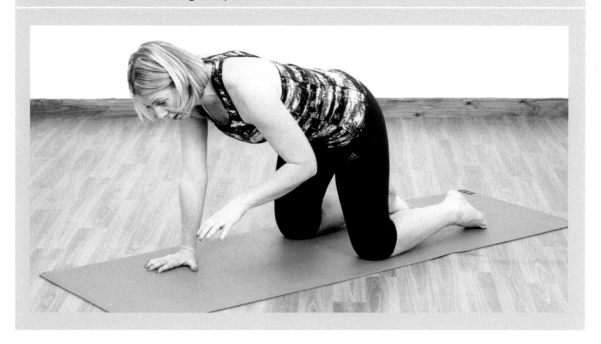

Purpose

To learn control of the four-point kneeling position while moving the limbs.

Preparation

Begin with the client in the box position, kneeling on all fours with their hands directly beneath their shoulders, knees beneath their hips. Their arms and upper legs should be vertical, their spine in its neutral position.

Action

Your client unloads their left arm by lifting the heel of their hand and then their fingers. They bend their elbow and lift their hand 5–10 cm from the floor maintaining horizontal alignment across their shoulders. Holding the upper position and replacing their hand on the ground, they re-establish their starting position before repeating the movement by lifting the right hand.

Tips

As they lift their hand your client's weight must be supported by their right hand and knees. You may find their upper body shifts towards the weight-bearing arm, but upper body alignment should remain intact. There is a tendency with this movement to dip down on the side of the bending arm and lose the horizontal alignment across the shoulder blades. This action imparts a rotation stress on the spine and moves the spine out of optimal alignment. Where this happens placing a book or pole across the shoulder blades enables your client to feel shoulder position more accurately.

Exercise 10.12 Threading the needle

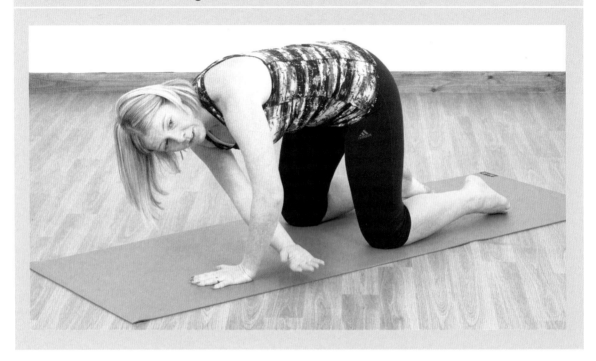

Purpose

To mobilise the spine to rotation while maintaining optimal spinal alignment in kneeling.

Preparation

Begin with the client kneeling in the box position with their hands beneath their shoulders and knees beneath their hips.

Action

The client performs the cat paw action (see p. 215) unloading the right hand. With their arm straight, they move it outwards and upwards (abduction and extension), keeping their hand in line with their shoulder. They should watch their hand as it goes upwards, to provide rotation through the whole length of the spine. Pause in the upper position and then draw the hand back down to the floor and then across the chest and between the left arm and left knee. Rest and repeat the action with the left arm.

Tips

The focus of this exercise is the spinal rotation. By watching the hand the client's attention is taken away from the spine towards the moving arm. Ensure that spinal alignment is maintained, as there is a tendency to hyperextend the spine as the arm moves backwards and to hyperflex it as it moves beneath the body. If they are unable to maintain a stable scapular position with their hand beneath their shoulder, move their hands forward by one hand length (giving 110° shoulder flexion rather than 90°).

Exercise 10.13 Clam

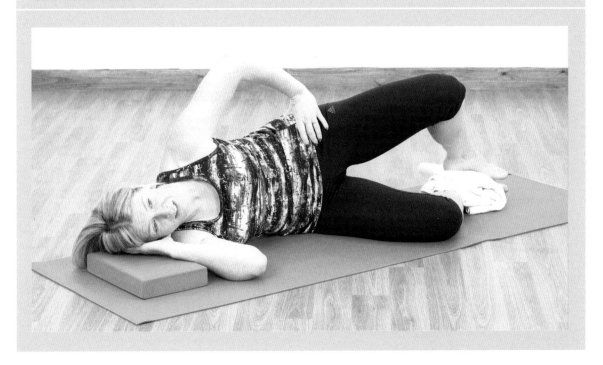

Purpose
To build endurance in the hip adductor muscles for maintenance of optimal alignment in single leg standing.

Preparation
Begin with the client lying on their side with knees bent to 90° and feet together. Place a folded towel between their feet for comfort.

Action
Your client should engage the gluteal muscles by visualising drawing their sitting bones together. Next they should exhale and lift their top knee upwards in an arching action, keeping their feet together, pause in the upper position and then inhale to lower under control.

Your client should then perform the same action as above, but begin with their feet 15–20 cm off the floor and keep them in this position as they lift their knee.

Tips
Your client should maintain alignment of the pelvis so that their hip bones remain stacked, avoiding leaning their pelvis forwards or backwards and imparting rotation on the lumbar spine.

Exercise 10.14 Toy soldier

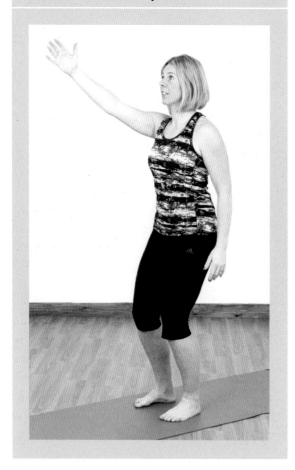

Purpose

To train scapulo-thoracic stability during free arm movement.

Preparation

Begin with the client standing with their feet hip-width apart (knees soft), arms by their sides, palms facing inwards.

Action

Focus on scapular stability by asking your client to engage their scapula muscles in a shoulder squeeze action performing a gentle downward (depression) and inward (adduction) movement with their scapulae. Tell them to inhale, and as they exhale reach their right arm forwards and upwards, so that it passes approximately 5–10 cm away from their ear, pausing in the upper position and then lowering their arm under control.

Focusing on scapular stability, your client should inhale, and as they exhale lift both arms forwards to the horizontal position (shoulder level) keeping their hands wider than body-width apart. They should keep their left arm in position, and raise their right arm overhead, then pause, and lower their right arm back to the horizontal position before repeating the action lifting their left arm. Breathing with this movement should mean exhaling as they reach overhead and inhaling as their arms lower to recover.

Focusing on scapular stability, the client should inhale and, as they exhale, lift both arms forwards and upwards above head height until they come level with their ears, before pausing and then inhaling to lower the arms with control.

Tips

The aim of this movement is to move the arms freely on a stable and well-aligned base. Get your client to focus on maintaining the distance between their shoulder and ear and avoiding any shrugging action (scapular elevation). In addition, the movement involves thoracic extension (sternal lift) but the abdominal muscles should remain engaged to avoid any rib flaring.

Exercise 10.15 Abdominal preparation

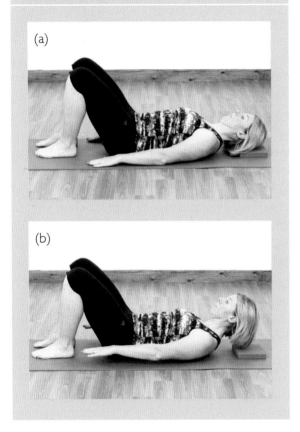

(a)

(b)

Purpose
To combine a pelvic floor contraction with deep and superficial abdominal muscle contraction.

Preparation
The client lies on their back with their knees bent, feet hip-width apart and flat. They should have their arms straight at the sides of their body, palms down.

Action
Instruct your client to breathe in and, as they breathe out, to perform a pelvic floor contraction and abdominal hollow. They should continue the action with a head nod (chin tuck) action and then lift their head from the mat into a neck curl. At the same time they should flex their thoracic spine, reaching their hands along the floor towards their outer ankle bones (lateral malleolus). As they flex their spine from the top downwards (cervical spine followed by thoracic spine) their spine forms a J-shape.

The action can be taken further by posteriorly tilting the pelvis to flex the spine upwards from below (i.e. pelvis followed by lumbar spine), to form a C-shape with the spine.

Tips
This action begins flexion of the whole spine into a C-curve. The movement involves contracting and shortening the abdominals by pulling the lower ribs towards the pubis. Where the abdominals are lengthened as a result of poor tone, obesity, pregnancy or post-surgical recovery, the available movement range will be quite small.

Definition
A head nod (also called chin tuck) action involves keeping the back of the head in contact with the floor and tucking the chin in to perform upper cervical flexion only. A neck curl involves lifting the head from the floor to perform flexion of the whole cervical spine (upper and lower regions).

Exercise 10.16 Seated roll back

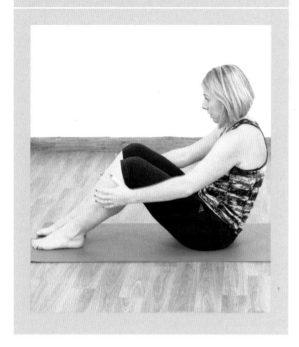

Purpose

To mobilise the spine into flexion, and strengthen and shorten the superficial abdominal muscles.

Preparation

Begin with your client sitting on the floor with their knees bent, feet hip-width apart and flat on the floor.

Action

Your client should hold onto the sides of their knees with their fingertips. They should inhale and then exhale and gradually take their body-weight backwards, forming a J-curve with their spine by flexing their cervical spine (chin tuck), then their thoracic spine (ribcage depression). At the same time they should flex their lumbar spine, posteriorly tilting their pelvis so their lumbar region rests flat on the mat and their spine forms a C-curve. Instruct them to support their upper bodyweight using their hands, and maintain the C-curve as they sit back up to recover.

The client should then begin with their hands 5–10 cm to the sides of their knees, palms facing inwards. Inhaling and then exhaling, they take their bodyweight backwards, forming a C-curve with their spine until their lumbar region rests flat on the mat. They then breathe in and maintain the C-curve in their spine as they sit back up to recover.

Next the client begins with their hands behind their head, supporting it lightly. They should inhale and then exhale and take their bodyweight backwards forming a C-curve with their spine until their lumbar region rests flat on the mat. Breathing in and maintaining the C-curve in their spine, they sit back up to recover.

Tips

This is an intense contraction of the abdominal muscles, so will limit diaphragmatic breathing. Focus the client's breathing into their side ribs (lateral costal breathing). For the last action, if their shoulder flexibility does not allow you to place the hands behind the neck, place the backs of the hands onto the forehead instead.

Exercise 10.17 Cat stretch

(a)

(b)

Purpose
To mobilise the whole spine into flexion and extension

Preparation
The client begins by kneeling on all fours with their hands beneath their shoulders and knees beneath their hips (box position).

Action
The client inhales, and as they exhale flexes their cervical spine (head nod followed by neck curl) and posteriorly tilts their pelvis. They continue the flexion to their thoracic spine, pressing their mid-back upwards and rounding it to form a C-shape. Next, they should pause in the flexed position and then inhale to return to the starting position.

Instruct your client to inhale and extend their cervical spine and anteriorly tilt their pelvis. They then continue the spinal extension action by lowering their abdomen and arching the whole of their spine to form a reverse C-shape.

Tips
This action must be maintained under muscle control throughout its whole sequence. Do not allow your client to build momentum, and encourage them to aim to move throughout the whole length of their spine vertebra by vertebra.

Exercise 10.18 Shell stretch

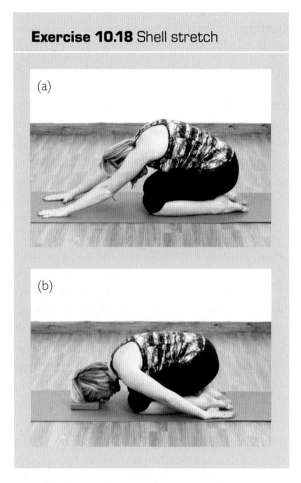

(a)

(b)

Purpose

To relax the spine into a supported semi-flexed position and maximally flex the hips.

Preparation

The client begins kneeling on all fours with knees hip distance apart, hands slightly in front of their shoulder line.

Action

The client sits back towards their ankles, keeping their hands in position. As they rest their buttocks onto their ankles, instruct them to relax their head and place their forehead onto the mat, before moving their arms to the sides of their body, palms upwards. They should relax in this position, focusing on lateral breathing.

Modify the position by getting your client to widen their knees to 1.5 hip-width and placing their toes closer together. They should sit back onto their heels so that the sides of their ribcage rest on their knees, but their breastbone passes between their knees. Next they must reach their arms forwards, placing their hands 1.5–2.0 times shoulder-width apart, palms downwards.

Tips

Action 1 rests the spine into a semi-flexed position. Action 2 allows the chest to drop lower and extends the thoracic spine, a position enforced by reaching the arms forwards. Action 2 is useful for clients who have a stiff and/or rounded (flexed) thoracic spine due to a kyphotic posture. In either action, if the head does not reach the floor with good cervical alignment, place the forehead on a folded towel or slim foam block. Also, in cases where knee flexion is limited, place a thick folded towel or blanket between the heels and buttocks.

Exercise 10.19 Rolling like a ball

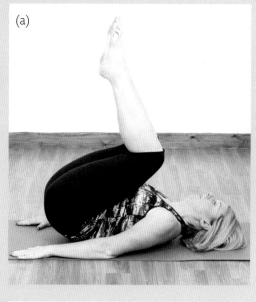

(a)

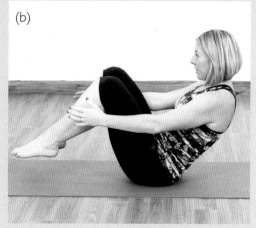

(b)

Purpose

To mobilise the spine into flexion and emphasise coordination and control of gross body movement.

Preparation

Begin with the client sitting with their knees bent and feet flat and together (crook sitting). They should bend (flex) their whole spine into a C-shape and reach their hands to the outside of their lower shins or ankles.

Action

Your client maintains a static C-shaped curve to their spine with their chin tucked in slightly, feet on the floor. Placing their hands on the ground by the sides of their hips, they should roll backwards, placing their arms on the mat, continuing the roll until their knees pass over their face. Reverse the action and roll forwards into the bent knee sitting position to recover.

The client begins sitting with their knees bent and feet flat on the floor, as in action 1. They should place their hands on the sides of their lower shins and lightly grip. Next they should keep their knees bent as they roll backwards through the full length of their spine to finish on their shoulders with their knees above their face, head resting on the mat. Reversing the action, they now roll backwards maintaining the C-shape in their spine to finish in the bent-knee sitting position.

Tips

This action requires control of momentum to roll through the full length of the spine. Make sure the client avoids falling back into the position and striking their head on the mat. Make sure they pause at the endpoint of each movement direction to avoid building too much momentum.

Exercise 10.20 Leg pull

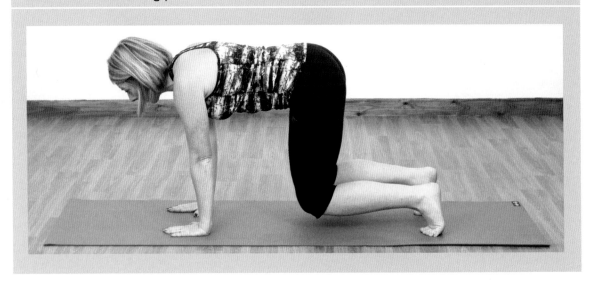

Purpose

To build scapula, thoracic and lumbar stability while enhancing upper-body strength.

Preparation

Begin with the client in a four point kneeling (box) position, with their hands slightly forwards of the shoulder line to give 110° shoulder flexion.

Action

The client should inhale to prepare and lean their bodyweight forwards over their hands as they lift their knees 2–3 cm above the floor. They should hover their knees in this position and then exhale to lower.

The client then places their hands on the floor 15–20 cm forwards of their shoulder line, in the four-point kneeling position. Talk them through stabilising their scapulae and taking their bodyweight forward to move their shoulders directly over their hands. At the same time get them to hover their knees above the floor, and then straighten their legs to form a straight line from their ear through their shoulders and hips to their ankles in a plank position.

The client performs the plank and then maintains the position. They should inhale to prepare, and as they exhale lift their right leg towards the horizontal keeping it straight. They then lower the leg, inhaling to recover. When they have re-established a good plank alignment, they should reverse the movement by raising their left leg to the horizontal.

Tips

Encourage your client to focus closely on maintaining alignment, keeping a neutral position of the lumbar and cervical spines at all times. Common errors include pressing the hips too far upwards (buttocks high), ballooning the abdominal muscles and lifting the head to give cervical extension. In addition make sure that their legs are straight but their knees do not hyperextend.

Exercise 10.21 Swimming from kneeling

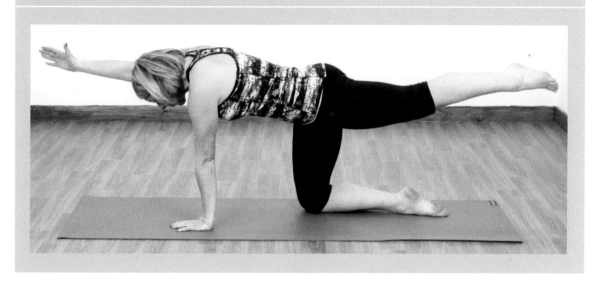

Purpose

To develop a high degree of lumbo-pelvic stabilisation with the spine in a gravity eliminated kneeling position.

Preparation

Begin with the client in a four-point kneeling or quadruped box position with their knees directly beneath their hips and hands directly beneath their shoulders.

Action

The client must gently perform the abdominal hollowing action and maintain a stable centre throughout the exercise. Instruct your client to inhale and, as they exhale, to lift their right arm forwards and upwards to an angle of 45° with the vertical, and at the same time slide their left leg backwards along the mat keeping their toes in contact with the mat surface. Next they should inhale, drawing their leg and arm back into the starting position to recover.

The client inhales and as they exhale simultaneously lifts their right arm forwards and upwards towards the horizontal and their left leg backwards and upwards towards the horizontal. Next they inhale and lower both their arm and their leg and repeat the movement using their right arm and left leg.

Tips

If your client finds it difficult to maintain scapular alignment with their hand directly beneath their shoulder in the box position, they may allow their hands to go 10 cm forwards so that they form approximately 110° of shoulder flexion. Their elbow joint should be just short of full extension (soft). Where balance in the four-point kneeling position is poor or your client requires full weight support of the spine, get them to practise swimming from lying (see p. 212) instead.

Exercise 10.22 The hundred

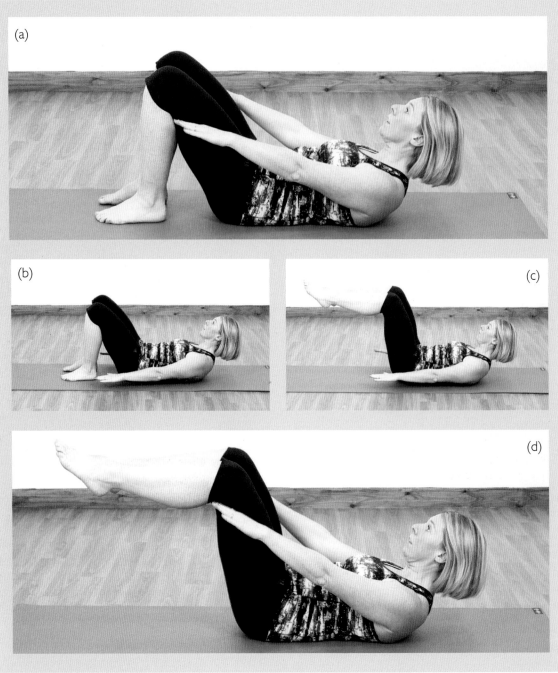

Purpose

To provide integrated activity and endurance of the superficial (GMS) and deep (SMS) abdominal muscles.

Preparation

Begin with the client lying on their back with their knees bent and feet flat and hip-width apart. Have them move to the imprint position, by activating their pelvic floor and abdominal hollowing. Get them to gently press their lumbar region towards (but not into) the floor. At the same time ask them to depress their ribcage to create the feeling of their ribs sliding downwards. They should place their arms at their sides, slightly away from their body, keeping them straight with their palms facing downwards.

Action

Have your client inhale, and as they exhale instruct them to maintain a light abdominal contraction and lift and lower their straight arms in a pulsing action. Then have them inhale for five arm movements and exhale for five.

The client performs action 1, and raises their right knee over their right hip, keeping the knee flexed to 90° (not pictured). Use the same timing as action 1, inhaling for five and exhaling for five. They then lower the leg so the foot is on the floor and repeat the sequence with the left leg.

Next, ask the client to perform action 1, but lift both legs (one at a time) so that the knees are above the hips, knees flexed to 90° so that the thigh bones (femur) are vertical and the shin bones (tibia) are horizontal. They should perform a pulsing action with the arms, using five movements to inhale and five to exhale, for a total of 10 breaths.

Lastly as a variation, the client could perform, but straightens the legs to 90° hip flexion and performs a pulsing action with the arms using five movements to inhale and five to exhale, for 10 breaths.

Tips

Although this action is designed to build abdominal endurance, the most important aspect is maintenance of good alignment. Common faults include allowing the abdominal wall to dome, allowing the lower rib cage to flare and losing alignment of the cervical spine by moving into a poking chin posture. If any of these faults occur stop the exercise and readjust your client's posture before continuing.

Exercise 10.23 Swandive

(a)

(b)

(c)

Purpose

To exercise the spinal extensor muscles with focus on the thoracic and lumbar spine, rather than lumbar spine alone.

Preparation

Begin with the client lying on their front with their arms bent, hands to the sides of their head (W position). They should allow their legs to relax with feet apart and ankles turned outwards to avoid a powerful contraction in the gluteals.

Action

Ask your client to press with their arms to raise their thoracic spine from the mat and lift their breastbone upwards and forwards. They should come to the forearm support position and broaden their shoulders, moving the scapulae downwards. They should keep their head aligned with their spine by performing a gentle chin tuck action and avoiding a poking chin posture.

From action 1, they client should lift their arms to hover them above the ground maintaining the lengthened body position and drawing their scapulae down.

Keeping their arms in the W position on the floor, the client should lift both legs back and upwards (hip extension), focusing on body length rather than height.

Instruct your client to combine actions 2 and 3 by lifting their chest from the mat with their arms. They should lower their chest and touch the floor with their forearms and, as they do so, lift their legs. Next, ask them to speed the movement up so they perform a controlled rocking action, lifting their legs and then chest, pivoting on their abdomen and maintaining the extended spine position.

Tips

Ensure that your client's spine extends through its full length and avoids any pinching in a single spinal segment (as this is evidence of hyperextension). The client must keep their abdominal muscles active throughout the movement. As they draw their scapulae down, make sure they maintain the distance between the scapulae and avoid adducting them forcibly. The scapula muscles should be active to stabilise the scapulae but not forcibly bracing them back and together, as with a military posture.

REFERENCES

Accident Compensation Corporation (2004) *New Zealand Acute Low Back Pain Guide.* Available at www.acc.co.nz, accessed June 2013.

Buer, N. and Linton, S. J. (2002) Fear-avoidance beliefs and catastrophising: occurrence and risk factor in back pain and ADL in the general population. *Pain* 99(3): 485–491.

Colloca, C.J., Hinrichs, R.N. (2005) The biomechanical and clinical significance of the lumbar erector spinae flexion-relaxation phenomenon: a review of literature. *Journal of Manipulative and Physiological Therapeutics* 28(8): 623–31.

Cramer, H., Lauche, R., Haller, H., Dobos, G. (2013) A systematic review and meta-analysis of yoga for low back pain. *Clinical journal of pain* 29(5): 450–60.

Demoulin, C., Vanderthommen M., Duysens, C. and Crielaard, J.-M. (2006) Spinal muscle evaluation using the Sorensen test: a critical appraisal of the literature. *Joint Bone Spine* 73: 43–50.

Descarreaux, M., Lafond, D., Jeffrey-Gauthier, R., Centomo, H., Cantin, V. (2008) Changes in the flexion relaxation response induced by lumbar muscle fatigue. *Musculoskeletal disorders* 9(10): 1471.

Groessl, E. J., Weingart, K. R., Johnson, N., Baxi, S. (2012) The benefits of yoga for women veterans with chronic low back pain. *Journal of alternative and complementary medicine* 18(9): 832–8.

Hicks, G. E., Fritz, J. M., Delitto, A. and McGill, S. M. (2005) Preliminary development of a clinical prediction rule for determining which patients with low back pain will respond to a stabilization exercise program. *Archives of Physical Medicine and Rehabilitation* 86:1753–62.

Key, J. (2010) *Back pain: a movement problem* (Churchill Livingstone, Edinburgh).

Krolner, B., Toft, B. and Nielsen, S. (1983) Physical exercise as a prophylaxis against involutional bone loss: a controlled trial. *Clinical science* 64: 541–546.

Naveen, K., Nagarathna, R., Nagendra, H. and Telles, S. (1997) Yoga breathing through a particular nostril increases spatial memory scores without lateralized effects. *Psychological Reports* 81: 555–561.

Norris, C. M. (2007) Weight training for Back Stability. In Liebenson, C. (ed.) *Rehabilitation of the Spine* (2nd edition). (Williams and Wilkins. Philadelphia, Pennsylvania).

Norris, C. M. (2008) *Resistance training for Core Strength* (Human Kinetics, Champaign, Illinois.) Chapter 14: Back Stability.

Norris, C. M. (2008) *Back Stability* (2nd edition) (Human Kinetics Champaign, Illinois).

Norris, C. M. and Mathews, M. (2008) The role of an integrated back stability program in patients with chronic low back pain. *Complementary Therapies in Clinical Practice* 14: 255–263.

Norris, C.M. (2011) *Managing Sports Injuries* (4th edition) (Churchill Livingstone, Edinburgh).

Page, P., Frank, C. C. and Lardner, R. (2010) *Assessment and treatment of muscle imbalance: the*

Janda approach (Human Kinetics, Champaign, Illinois).

Pomidori, L., Campigotto, F., Amatya, T., Bernardi, L. (2009) Efficacy and Tolerability of Yoga Breathing in Patients With Chronic Obstructive Pulmonary Disease. *Journal of Cardiopulmonary Rehabilitation & Prevention* 29(2): 133–137.

Sengupta, P. (2012) Health impacts of yoga and pranayama: a state-of-the-art review. *International journal of preventive medicine* 3(7): 444–458.

Sherman, K. J., Cherkin, D. C., Erro, J. *et al* (2005) Comparing yoga, exercise and a self care book for chronic low back pain: a randomised controlled trial. *Annals of internal medicine* 143: 849–856.

Shiri, R., Solovieva, S. *et al* (2012) The role of obesity and physical activity in non-specific and radiating low back pain: the young Finns study. *Seminars in arthritis and rheumatism* 42(6): 640–650.

Singh, V., Wisniewski, A., Britton J. and Tattersfield, A. (1990) Effect of yoga breathing exercises (pranayama) on airway reactivity in subjects with asthma. *Lancet* 335(9) 1381–1383.

Singleton, M. (2010) *Yoga body: the origins of modern posture practice* (Oxford University Press).

Smith, E. I., Smith, P. E. and Ensign, C. J. (1984) Bone involutional decrease in exercising middle aged women. *Calcified tissue international,* 36(1): 129–138.

Symonds, T. L., Burton, A. K., Tillotson, K. M. and Main, C. J., (1996) Do attitudes and beliefs influence work loss due to low back trouble? *Occupational Medicine* 46(1): 25–32.

Tekur, P., Singphow, C., Ramarao Nagendra, H. and Raghuram, R. (2008) Effect of short-term intensive yoga program on pain, functional disability and spinal flexibility in chronic low back pain: a randomized control study. *Journal of Alternative and Complementary Medicine* 14(6) 637–644.

Tilbrook, H. E., Cox, H., Hewitt, C. E., Chuang L.-H. *et al* (2011) Yoga for chronic low back pain: a randomised trial. *Annals of Internal Medicine* November.

Waddell, G., Somerville, D., Henderson, I, Newton, M. and Main, C. J. (1993) A fear avoidance beliefs questionnaire (FABQ) and the role of fear avoidance beliefs in chronic low back pain and disability. *Pain* 52: pp. 157–168.

Waddell, G. (2004) *The back pain revolution* (Churchill Livingstone, Edinburgh). Chapter 12: 'Beliefs about back pain'.

Williams, K., Abildso, C., Steinberg, L. *et al* (2009) Evaluating the effectiveness and efficacy of Iyengar yoga therapy on chronic low back pain. *Spine* 34(19): 2066–2076.

Williams, M. and Penman, D. (2011) *Mindfulness* (Piatkus, London).

INDEX